S0-AJV-212

THE EASY ACID REFLUX COOKBOOK

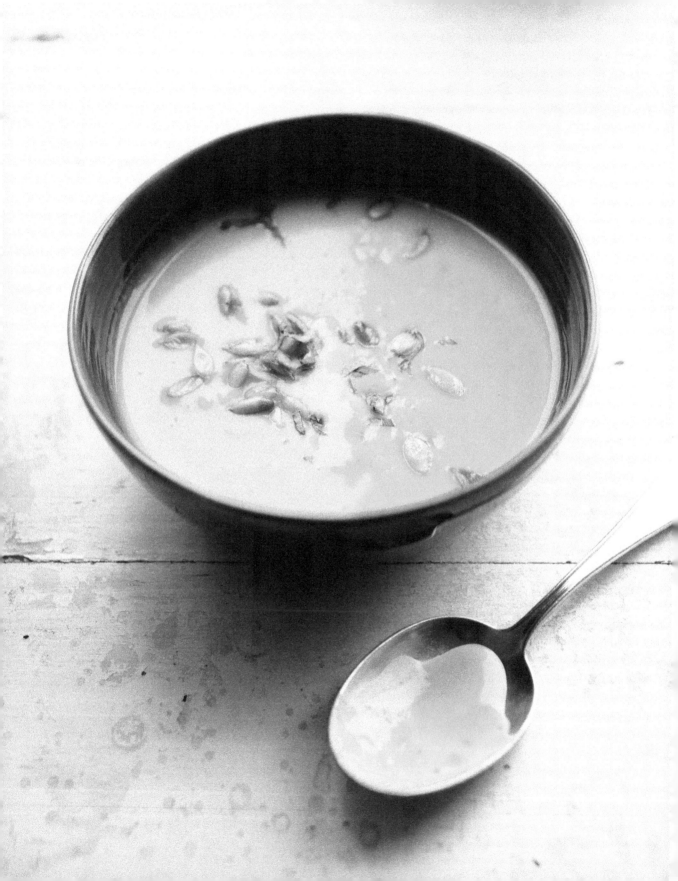

THE easy ACID REFLUX COOKBOOK

Comforting 30-Minute Recipes to Soothe GERD & LPR

KAREN FRAZIER

ROCKRIDGE
PRESS

*For Jim, and for anyone else
who suffers from GERD*

Copyright © 2017 by Rockridge Press, Berkeley, California

No part of this publication may be reproduced, stored in a retrieval system, or transmitted in any form or by any means, electronic, mechanical, photocopying, recording, scanning, or otherwise, except as permitted under Sections 107 or 108 of the 1976 US Copyright Act, without the prior written permission of the Publisher. Requests to the Publisher for permission should be addressed to the Permissions Department, Rockridge Press, 918 Parker St, Suite A-12, Berkeley, CA 94710.

Limit of Liability/Disclaimer of Warranty: The Publisher and the author make no representations or warranties with respect to the accuracy or completeness of the contents of this work and specifically disclaim all warranties, including without limitation warranties of fitness for a particular purpose. No warranty may be created or extended by sales or promotional materials. The advice and strategies contained herein may not be suitable for every situation. This work is sold with the understanding that the Publisher is not engaged in rendering medical, legal, or other professional advice or services. If professional assistance is required, the services of a competent professional person should be sought. Neither the Publisher nor the author shall be liable for damages arising herefrom. The fact that an individual, organization, or website is referred to in this work as a citation and/or potential source of further information does not mean that the author or the Publisher endorses the information the individual, organization, or website may provide or recommendations they/it may make. Further, readers should be aware that websites listed in this work may have changed or disappeared between when this work was written and when it is read.

For general information on our other products and services or to obtain technical support, please contact our Customer Care Department within the United States at (866) 744-2665, or outside the United States at (510) 253-0500.

Rockridge Press publishes its books in a variety of electronic and print formats. Some content that appears in print may not be available in electronic books, and vice versa.

TRADEMARKS: Rockridge Press and the Rockridge Press logo are trademarks or registered trademarks of Callisto Media Inc., and/or its affiliates, in the United States and other countries, and may not be used without written permission. All other trademarks are the property of their respective owners. Rockridge Press is not associated with any product or vendor mentioned in this book.

Front cover photography © Con Poulos/Offset

Interior photography © Stocksy/J.R. Photography, p.2 (Pumpkin Soup recipe, p.6); Stockfood/Valerie Janssen, p.6; Stocksy/Tatjana Ristanic, p.10; Stockfood/Marie José Jarry, p.30; Con Poulos/Offset, p.44; Stockfood/Yvonne Duivenvoorden, p.62; Stockfood/People Pictures, p.78; Stockfood/Rua Castilho, p.94; Stockfood/People Pictures, p.112; Stockfood/Gräfe & Unzer Verlag/Jörn Rynio, p.130; Stockfood/Sporrer/Skowronek, p.148

Back cover photography © Stockfood/Sporrer/Skowronek; StockFood/Rua Castilho; Stocksy/J.R. PHOTOGRAPHY; Stockfood/People Pictures

ISBN: Print 978-1-62315-874-3
eBook 978-1-62315-875-0

GERD-Friendly Versions of Your Favorite Foods

Just because you have acid reflux doesn't mean you can't eat some of your favorite comfort foods. While many comfort foods are high in fat or contain acidic or other ingredients that might aggravate GERD (gastro-esophageal reflux disease), with a few simple adjustments you still can enjoy many of your favorite foods.

The foods in this book are low in fat and acid, and though the portions may be smaller, they'll satisfy your cravings for comforting, delicious, flavorful foods, which is the right recipe for keeping you on track as you eat to avoid triggering acid reflux flare-ups.

You'll find plenty of satisfying and delicious recipes here, including GERD-friendly versions of the classic comfort foods you love.

MAC 'N' CHEESE (page 57) made in single-serving portions with much less fat than the traditional version. Eating a small portion will give you all the flavor you want, without the heartburn.

BURGERS are typically heartburn waiting to happen. The leaned-down, smaller-portion Turkey Sliders (page 99) give you the burger experience with a lovely umami sauce, without any of the acid reflux you might expect.

PIZZA gets a GERD makeover with a flavorful white sauce and low-fat toppings that truly taste mouthwatering. Try Mini Pizzas with Canadian Bacon and White Sauce (page 105) or Mini Pizzas with Spinach and White Sauce (page 80).

POTATO CHIPS don't have to go by the wayside. Enjoy lightly salty, crispy Baked Potato Chips (page 53) instead.

ENJOY POTATO SALAD (page 67) with all the flavor of the original, minus the fat and GERD-triggering ingredients.

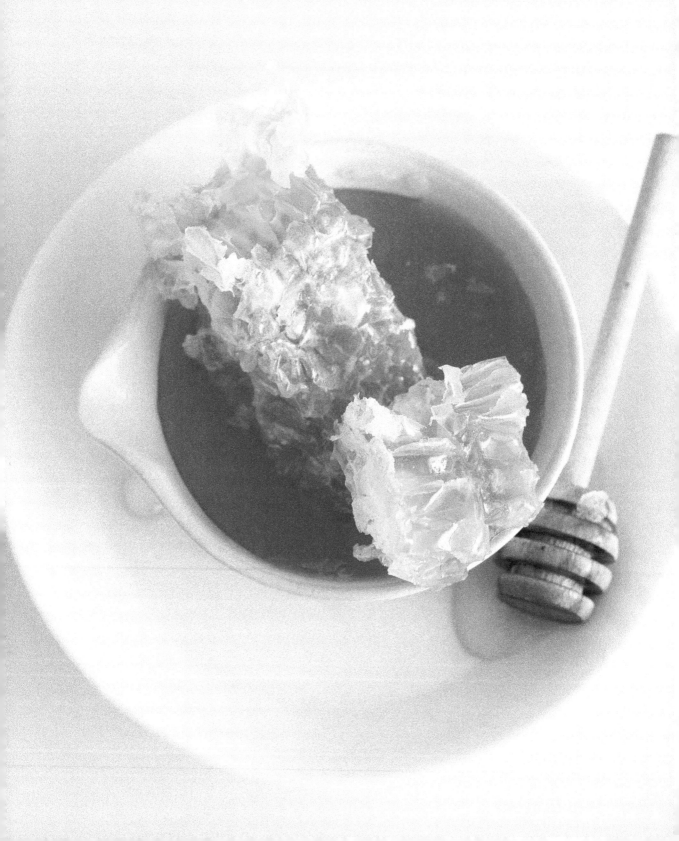

Contents

For several years, I was almost certain I would have to stop eating altogether. Shortly after eating anything, I suffered the most intense pain. Sometimes, the pain doubled me over. Often, it disturbed my sleep and made it difficult to pursue simple activities because I felt terrible. While medications helped initially, eventually I needed to switch to stronger versions, and then to different types altogether to keep my acid reflux in check. It was no way to live.

Unfortunately, the medications often came with unwanted side effects and could do harm if I took them long term. I needed another solution, so I started exploring dietary options to control my symptoms.

This was daunting—the dietary approach seemed such a drastic change from how I usually ate. Because I have other food sensitivities and restrictions as well (I am allergic to dairy products and I have celiac disease, which means I can't tolerate gluten), I knew if I ever wanted to feel better and get my life back, I needed to change my diet. So I started creating recipes for delicious foods I could substitute for those that were aggravating my GERD (gastroesophageal reflux disease).

As I developed recipes, it got easier to change the way I ate to support my physical health. Now, eating to control my health conditions, including GERD, is second nature. I haven't suffered from acid reflux symptoms in more than two years, and I have my life back.

Acid reflux is surprisingly common. According to a literature review published in the journal *Gut*, GERD is symptomatic in 10 to 20 percent of the population, and Healthline notes that at least 60 percent of the population will experience a bout of acid reflux within a 12-month period, while 20 to 30 percent notice weekly symptoms. Although many believe GERD is a disease that primarily affects elderly populations, it can occur in people of all ages. So if you're suffering from bouts of acid reflux, know that you aren't alone. The symptoms can range from mild to debilitating, and they can affect multiple areas of your life.

You may be feeling overwhelmed as you look into changing your diet and lifestyle to help eliminate your symptoms. Making major dietary and lifestyle changes can feel stressful for many reasons.

There's a big learning curve. Learning about eating for a specific health condition is time consuming if you do the research yourself, and it's difficult to determine good information from bad.

Additional conditions may complicate your dietary picture. If you're like me (and many others), acid reflux isn't the only issue you're facing. This may make it difficult to determine which foods will help or harm other health conditions you may have.

Cravings make it difficult to stick to a restrictive diet. If you have to give up many of the foods you love, it is difficult to sustain a restrictive diet for life.

Cooking for yourself takes time. For many people, time is one of the biggest issues in why they continue to eat as they do, in spite of how it affects their health. Cooking for yourself can be time consuming.

This book is designed to solve all of these problems.

1. **You won't need to do the research yourself.** This book contains all the information you need about dietary and lifestyle choices you can make to improve your symptoms. All information is based on the latest scientific and medical findings for controlling acid reflux.

2. **Recipes are labeled for many dietary restrictions.** Each recipe is clearly labeled so you can determine which ones work with specific health conditions (like IBS or diabetes), or for special diets like the paleo diet or a low-carb diet.

3. **The rich flavors help satisfy cravings.** The recipes are delicious and make excellent substitutes for some of your favorite comfort foods, but they do so in an acid reflux–friendly manner, so you'll be less likely to give in to cravings.

4. **You can make quick meals ahead of time.** Recipes take 30 minutes or less, and you can make and freeze many of them ahead of time for quick meals on the go. Likewise, the recipes don't contain any special or hard-to-find ingredients, don't require any specialized equipment, and the instructions are clear and easy to follow.

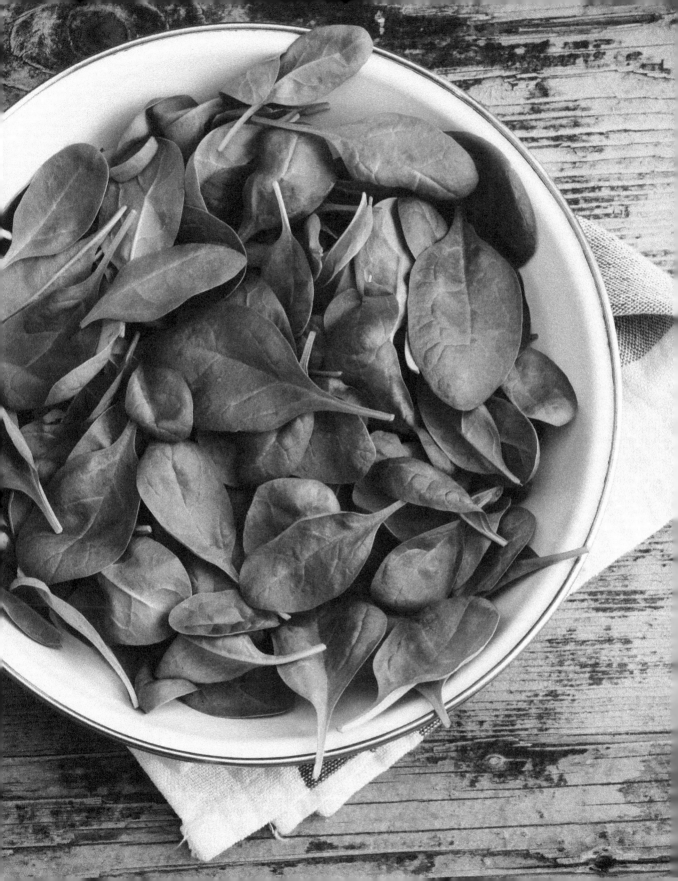

ONE

Managing Acid Reflux through Diet

It is possible to manage your acid reflux symptoms by making dietary changes. There are numerous changes, big and small, you can make to the way you eat to help control your symptoms, as well as certain ingredients to avoid that trigger these symptoms. Knowing and following these dietary "rules" for acid reflux can make a huge difference in the way you eat and in the way you feel.

The Causes of Heartburn

You'll hear people call similar symptoms by different names: heartburn, acid reflux, indigestion, or GERD. Really, they are all degrees of the same condition. For example, GERD is the term used when acid reflux, indigestion, or heartburn is chronic and causing damage to the alimentary canal (food's pathway through the body from entry to exit). When the acid makes its way into the throat, the condition is called laryngo-pharyngeal reflux, or LPR.

Weakened Lower Esophageal Sphincter

All of these conditions arise from the same cause, according to the Mayo Clinic. Heartburn happens when stomach acid or bile backs up into the esophagus. To understand how this happens, you first need to recognize what occurs every time you swallow food or drink. When you swallow, the food goes down your esophagus and into your stomach. As it passes through into your stomach, a group of muscles called the lower esophageal sphincter (LES) closes, keeping the food in your stomach as digestion begins.

Sometimes, the LES grows weak and no longer closes around the esophagus after food or drink passes through. When this happens, acid from the stomach can pass through the LES and up into the esophagus, causing discomfort, irritation, inflammation, and eventually, even damage. This is what causes the discomfort associated with acid reflux.

These things weaken the LES:

- Consumption of alcoholic beverages
- Consumption of caffeinated beverages including coffee, tea, and energy drinks
- Tobacco use
- Ingestion of certain foods known to weaken the LES such as chocolate, mint, and peppers

Increased Acid Production

With a weakened LES, excessive acid production can be bad news. Anything that increases the production of stomach acid will increase the likelihood of acid reflux. These are some things to avoid:

- Eating acidic foods such as vinegar, citrus fruits, and pineapple
- Taking certain medications such as ibuprofen, aspirin, and antibiotics
- Overusing acid-suppressing medications such as proton pump inhibitors, which can cause rebound acid production when you stop taking them

Age

As people age, they generally lose muscle tone unless effort is made to preserve it, according to the US National Library of Medicine. Since the LES is made up of muscles, there may be a natural loss of tone as you age, which may contribute to acid reflux.

Certain Medications

Many medications can cause a weakening of the LES and contribute to GERD and LPR, according to Health.com. These are some of the medications:

- Bisphosphonates, which are osteoporosis medications
- Calcium channel blockers, typically used as blood pressure medication
- Sedatives and sleeping pills, which relax the LES
- Tricyclic antidepressants, such as amitriptyline, which slow the release of stomach contents, increasing intra-abdominal pressure

Increased Intra-Abdominal Pressure

Likewise, increased pressure in the abdominal region may exert excessive force on the LES, causing it to weaken and allowing acid to leak into the esophagus. When you temporarily increase intra-abdominal pressure (IAP), it can force acid up and through a weakened LES, causing symptoms. These things may increase IAP:

- Consumption of carbonated beverages
- Overeating or eating large portions
- Excessive weight gain or obesity, particularly in the abdominal region
- Consuming foods such as peppers, onions, and other fatty foods that cause gas, which increases pressure in the abdomen

- Bending or lying down shortly after eating
- Pregnancy
- Hiatal hernia, which occurs when part of the stomach pushes through an opening in the diaphragm into the chest cavity

Bacteria

According to functional medicine specialist Chris Kresser, bacterial overgrowth may also contribute to GERD by causing carbohydrate malabsorption, leading to gas and increased IAP. While this is a relatively new theory, Kresser and others suggest there may be a link between irritable bowel syndrome (IBS) and GERD, which may suggest that a certain category of poorly digested carbohydrates, called FODMAPs, may also contribute to GERD in certain cases because gas increases IAP. Bacterial issues in the gut may include small intestinal bacterial overgrowth and *H. pylori* infection.

Stress

A 2013 Korean study established that stress is also associated with acid reflux. While the mechanism behind stress and increased symptoms of acid reflux is poorly understood, Health.com notes researchers found that stress doesn't increase acid production, result in IAP, or weaken the LES. Instead, they hypothesize stress may either affect hormones in the stomach that block acid, or it may affect the brain in a way that causes you to perceive the discomfort associated with acid reflux more acutely.

The Relationship Between Food & Symptoms

You probably know, or possibly have experienced yourself, that eating certain foods can aggravate indigestion. Perhaps you ate a rich chocolate torte before bedtime and woke up several hours later with a burning in your chest and throat, or maybe a spicy dinner created the need to take antacids a few hours later. Many people have had such experiences and understand that, at least occasionally, eating some foods causes heartburn.

What you may not realize, however, is just how strong a connection there is between the foods you eat and acid reflux, GERD, and LPR. As discussed in the previous sections, there are three primary ways food can trigger GERD and its variants:

- It can weaken the LES.
- It can increase acidity in the stomach.
- It can increase IAP.

Acidity & Alkalinity

All substances have the property of pH, which measures the degree of acidity or alkalinity (or neutrality). If you recall basic high school chemistry, the higher the pH of something, the more alkaline it is. The lower the pH, the more acidic it is. A pH of 7 indicates the substance is neutral—that is, neither acidic nor basic. Likewise, you likely learned adding an alkaline substance to an acidic one neutralizes the acidity.

This principle also holds true with food. If you have a condition related to high acidity in your stomach, such as acid reflux and its variants, adding acidic foods to that system will make it even more acidic. Adding alkaline foods will help neutralize the acids.

Many people seek to neutralize the acids in their stomach with antacids, which are powerful alkaline substances that may neutralize stomach acid. However, the International Foundation for Functional Gastrointestinal Disorders (IFFGD) notes that although these substances are fast acting, they are also short-term, temporary solutions that may come with their own issues, such as causing rebound acidity (an increase in stomach acidity in response to taking them), as well as other unwanted side effects.

However, eating alkaline foods doesn't come with these same risks. Therefore, for permanent relief of acid reflux without side effects, your best bet is to choose alkaline foods and minimize acidic foods.

Food Allergies, Sensitivities, & Intolerances

As I revamped the way I ate, I discovered that one of my biggest acid reflux triggers was related to my food intolerances. What I discovered was that when I consumed a food to which I was intolerant, I was far more likely to develop acid reflux than when I did not. That's because food allergies and intolerances affect your body's ability to digest the foods you eat. Consuming them may cause issues that lead to increased IAP because they may

- delay the emptying of stomach contents.
- cause poor or incomplete digestion.
- cause bloating and gas.
- cause changes in gut bacteria (the gut microbiome).
- cause a condition with symptoms that overlap those of acid reflux.

People may be intolerant, sensitive, or allergic to several common foods or ingredients.

GLUTEN

Gluten is a protein found in wheat, rye, and barley. According to BeyondCeliac.org, about 1 percent of the population has celiac disease, an autoimmune form of gluten intolerance in which sufferers can't process even trace amounts of gluten. However, this number may be higher, as experts estimate about 83 percent of Americans with celiac disease remain undiagnosed or misdiagnosed. The organization further estimates about 18 million Americans don't have celiac disease, but they still have a gluten intolerance called non-celiac gluten sensitivity. Studies, including one published in the *Scandinavian Journal of Gastroenterology* in 2009, note a strong link between ingestion of gluten in intolerant individuals and acid reflux events. In these individuals with both a gluten intolerance (or celiac disease) and acid reflux, avoiding gluten is incredibly important to managing both conditions.

DAIRY PRODUCTS

For people with intolerance to dairy products (commonly arising from intolerance to the milk sugar lactose, or from an allergy to dairy's primary protein casein) GERD is often a co-occurring condition, according to Healthline. This isn't necessarily because dairy products cause GERD by themselves, but rather because intolerances can cause gas that increases IAP. It's important to avoid dairy if you are intolerant to it, especially if you are also trying to control acid reflux.

FODMAPS

Some people are sensitive to a certain category of poorly digested carbohydrates called FODMAPs. FODMAPs, or fermentable oligosaccharides, disaccharides, monosaccharides, and polyols, are carbohydrates that naturally occur in many foods, ranging from fruit and milk to grains and beans. For people with FODMAP sensitivity, which often manifests as IBS, eating these carbohydrates can cause a whole host of gastrointestinal symptoms including gas, bloating, delayed stomach emptying, and constipation, all of which can increase IAP and contribute to GERD. If you've been diagnosed with IBS, or other bowel diseases like Crohn's disease, inflammatory bowel disease (IBD), or colitis, you may be sensitive to FODMAPs in your diet. For more information about FODMAPs and how to avoid them, visit the Monash University Low FODMAP Diet for IBS (see Resources, page 179).

Avoiding Acid Reflux on Specific Diets

As healthcare professionals continue to discover how much the food you eat affects your health, more and more people are on specialized diets to help them control health conditions. The recipes in this book contain labels for people on specialized diets to help you know which foods will fit within your meal plan. The labels are as follows:

ALKALINE Recipes with this label contain primarily alkaline ingredients and have an overall alkaline pH to help reduce acid.

GLUTEN-FREE These recipes are perfect for people with celiac disease or non-celiac gluten sensitivity, as well as anyone who wishes to minimize the amount of gluten consumed.

LOW-CARB Recipes with this label will have 10 or fewer net grams of carbohydrates per serving, so they're great for people trying to control diabetes or lose weight with a low-carb diet.

LOW-FODMAP These recipes won't exacerbate IBS or IBD, and will help eliminate gassiness in people who process this type of carbohydrate poorly.

PALEO Paleo dieters "eat like cavemen." That is, they don't eat any processed foods and prefer to eat natural single-ingredient foods including meat, poultry, fish, eggs, vegetables, fruits, nuts, and seeds. Paleo diets are semi-low-carb diets, and many autoimmune protocols follow some version of the paleo diet. These recipes may be a great choice if you have an autoimmune disease.

VEGAN Vegan recipes contain no animal products at all.

VEGETARIAN Vegetarian recipes contain no animal products with the exception of dairy, eggs, and honey.

OTHER FOODS

It should also be noted that food allergies can create symptoms that appear to be acid reflux, but may actually be a condition called eosinophilic esophagitis (EE). According to the Mayo Clinic, EE occurs when white blood cells build up in the esophagus and become symptomatic. While EE occurs due to acid reflux, it has other causes as well, including being a reaction to consuming foods to which you are allergic. The resultant inflammation can cause a host of symptoms similar to GERD (or overlapping with it) that include difficulty swallowing, chest pain that doesn't respond to antacids, persistent heartburn, and regurgitation.

If you have GERD symptoms that don't respond (or don't respond as well as you hope) to GERD medications or an acid reflux diet, you may have EE associated with food or substance allergies. Common food allergens that may contribute to EE include the most common allergens—wheat, fish, shellfish, peanuts, tree nuts, dairy, and eggs—and less common allergies to foods. If you suspect food allergies are contributing to your symptoms, talk to your doctor about being tested.

RECIPE ADAPTATION

Because food intolerances, sensitivities, and allergies may be an issue for some, the recipes in this book have been adapted in the following ways:

- Where possible, substitution tips are offered for common allergens
- Labels are provided to help you determine whether a recipe suits your specific needs
- Low-FODMAP recipes are labeled

Likewise, you can adapt many of this book's recipes to meet your own individual dietary needs.

A Diet & Lifestyle Free of Acid Reflux

As you read the previous section, you probably began to develop an understanding of how you might modify your lifestyle and diet as you seek to cure your acid reflux. Now let's take those recommendations further, to truly change the way you eat and live to free yourself of those often-debilitating symptoms.

Avoid Foods or Substances That Weaken Your LES

If your LES is already weakened, eating foods that weaken it further can add to your symptoms, creating a downward spiral. There are many foods and substances that weaken your LES:

- Alcohol
- Caffeine
- Chocolate
- Citrus juice
- Fried foods
- Garlic
- High-fat foods
- Onions
- Peppermint
- Peppers
- Tomatoes

Avoid Foods or Substances That Increase Acidity

Acidic foods (see Appendix A, page 168) create more acid that can escape through a weakened LES, so it's important to avoid them. Here is a quick list of such foods:

- Alcohol
- Cashews
- Citrus fruits
- Coffee
- Dairy products
- Pasta
- Peanuts
- Pecans
- Pineapple
- Pistachios
- Processed grains
- Tomatoes
- Walnuts

Eat More Alkaline Foods

Consuming alkaline foods (see Appendix A, page 168) can help neutralize the acidity in your stomach, and, with less acid to escape through the LES, you will experience fewer symptoms. There are numerous alkaline foods:

- Fish and shellfish
- Fruits, except citrus and pineapple
- Lean meats
- Lean poultry
- Low-fat dairy
- Vegetables
- Whole grains

Avoid Foods That May Increase IAP

When you eat foods that increase IAP, you heighten the chances that acid will find its way in the wrong direction through the LES. These foods may increase IAP:

- Carbonated beverages
- Foods high in FODMAPs, if you are intolerant to them
- Gassy foods such as sugar alcohols

Eat Small Meals

Large meals increase IAP, which can aggravate symptoms. Opt for six small meals daily, and try to eat at least 90 percent of your food before 6 p.m.

Stop Eating at Least Four Hours Before Bedtime

Lying down with a full stomach does two things: it increases IAP, and puts you in a position that allows stomach contents to move easily upward through the LES. Give your food time to digest. Stop eating four hours before bedtime and you'll be less likely to have nighttime GERD symptoms.

Wear Loose Clothing

Tight clothing can also increase IAP, so loose, easy-fitting clothing can help minimize the chances you'll have flare-ups during the day.

If You're Overweight, Lose Weight

Obesity, particularly around the middle, can increase IAP and weaken the LES. Therefore, if GERD is an issue, losing weight can help.

Minimize Fat in Foods

In her book, *Dr. Koufman's Acid Reflux Diet*, Dr. Jamie Koufman notes fried and fatty foods are the single biggest trigger of acid reflux symptoms. This is because consuming high levels of fat relaxes the LES. Therefore, eating lean foods and avoiding fried and fatty foods can help minimize symptoms.

Watch What (and When) You Drink

Alcohol, soda, and caffeinated beverages can all trigger acid reflux, but even drinking too much water at inopportune times can be an issue. Avoid drinking large amounts of any beverage with meals, as this will also increase IAP. Instead, drink plenty of water to stay hydrated, but space it throughout the day to keep your stomach from overfilling and causing acid to splash up into the esophagus.

Emergency Help for Flare-Ups

Sometimes, even in spite of your best efforts, you may experience a flare-up of your acid reflux symptoms. Don't panic! Try to make reaching for an antacid your last resort. Instead, first try any of the following to soothe and manage your symptoms.

DRINK GINGER TEA

According to medical researcher, biochemist, and chiropractor Dr. David Williams, ginger is an effective remedy for acid reflux. So if you experience a flare-up, sip on a simple ginger tea. Steep one tablespoon of grated fresh ginger in hot water for 10 minutes. Strain and sip the tea.

CHEW GUM

Dr. Williams also recommends chewing gum (be sure it isn't mint!). Chewing gum increases saliva production, and saliva contains a substance that soothes the esophagus to help stop the burning.

DRINK ALOE VERA JUICE

Aloe vera juice may also help soothe heartburn flare-ups. A study published in the *Journal of Traditional Chinese Medicine* showed that consuming the juice alleviated symptoms and caused no side effects or rebound acidity. You can find aloe vera juice at your local health food store.

CHEW A FEW BASIL LEAVES

Natural News notes that chewing basil may help calm heartburn as well. It works by soothing the burning in the esophagus. You can buy or grow basil, or try drinking a premade (caffeine-free) basil tea.

IF YOU'RE IN BED, GET UP OR RAISE THE HEAD OF YOUR BED

If you have an acid reflux sneak attack when sleeping, get up and sit or stand for a while to stop the acid from splashing through your LES. You can also raise the head of your bed with blocks, books, or bedstands so your head is elevated above your feet, or prop up your upper body with pillows.

Food Tables

The following are helpful summaries of foods to avoid in order to improve your symptoms, as well as foods to consume in moderation, and foods you can enjoy without worrying they will trigger a flare-up.

AVOID THESE FOODS

FOOD OR FOOD GROUP	NOTEWORTHY INFORMATION
Alcoholic beverages	Relaxes LES
Caffeine	Stimulant; relaxes LES
Carbonated beverages	Acidic; increases abdominal pressure
Chiles, peppers, hot sauce	Known reflux triggers
Chocolate	Stimulant; known reflux cause
Citrus fruits and juices	Acidic
Cream sauces	High in fat
Dairy, full-fat or medium-fat (2 percent)	Avoid high-fat dairy such as butter, cheese, whole milk, full-fat yogurt or sour cream, and cream—if you use, use sparingly
Fried foods	Single largest trigger of heartburn and reflux
Fruit	Acidic fruits, fruits not noted on other lists, pineapple, citrus
Garlic	Known reflux trigger
Herbal or regular tea	Known reflux trigger
Margarine, shortening	High in fat and made with unnatural ingredients
Meat, beef	Avoid cuts higher than 15 percent fat
Meat, pork	Avoid all but the leanest cuts
Mint	Known reflux trigger
Onion	Known reflux trigger
Pepper, green bell	Known reflux trigger
Spicy food	Known reflux trigger

CONSUME WITH CAUTION

FOOD OR FOOD GROUP	NOTEWORTHY INFORMATION
Apple, green	Acidic; may cause problems for some people—eat red instead or avoid altogether if sensitive to FODMAPs
Artificial sweeteners	Limit to 1 to 2 teaspoons per day
Butter	Less than 2 teaspoons per day
Chamomile tea	1 cup per day or less
Cheese, Parmesan or sharp Cheddar only (full-fat)	Limit to 2 tablespoons per day or less; use primarily as flavoring—avoid if sensitive to dairy or FODMAPs
Coffee, decaffeinated	1 cup per day or less
Cucumber	May trigger reflux in some people
FODMAPs	Minimize or avoid if sensitive to FODMAPs or you have IBS
Mustard, Dijon	Less than 1 tablespoon per day for flavoring—if gluten sensitive, read label to make sure it doesn't contain wheat
Pepper, black	May trigger reflux in some people; use only very small amounts—one shake of the pepper shaker
Peppers, red bell	Less than ¼ pepper per day
Raisins	Don't eat by themselves; eat only in conjunction with whole grains, which will absorb some of the acid; limit to less than 2 tablespoons per day
Sesame seeds	1 tablespoon per day or less for flavor
Tomatoes	May trigger reflux in some people; use a small amount for flavoring, but eat in conjunction with starchy foods to blunt the effects; less than 2 tablespoons of tomato sauce per day
Vinaigrette	1 tablespoon per day or less

ENJOY WITH GUSTO

FOOD OR FOOD GROUP	NOTEWORTHY INFORMATION
Agave nectar	Low-glycemic sweetener adds flavor—avoid if sensitive to FODMAPs
Apple, red	Fuji, Red Delicious; four or fewer per week—avoid if sensitive to FODMAPs
Avocado	Excellent source of fiber and vitamins; great stand-in for high-fat dairy in salad dressing—avoid if sensitive to FODMAPs
Banana	A very small number of people may be sensitive, so if it is a trigger for you, avoid it
Beef, extra-lean cuts	Less than 15 percent fat
Berries	Great alkaline way to add flavor
Breads and muffins	Low-fat, nonfruit versions
Celery	Helps control appetite
Cereal	Whole-grain—avoid wheat, barley, oats if sensitive to gluten
Cheese	Nonfat—avoid if sensitive to FODMAPs
Citrus zest	Citrus flavor without the acid
Corn	All kinds, including cornmeal—avoid if sensitive to FODMAPs
Eggs	Four per day or fewer
Fennel	Improves stomach digestive function
Fish and shellfish	Baked, broiled, steamed, or grilled, but not fried
Fish sauce	Great way to add umami flavor
Ginger	Fresh or ground
Grains, whole	Starchy; absorb acid—be careful if sensitive to gluten or FODMAPs
Herbs and spices	All but peppers, chiles, and mint
Honey	Good for soothing heartburn—avoid if sensitive to FODMAPs
Legumes	Chickpeas, beans, peas, etc.

FOOD OR FOOD GROUP	NOTEWORTHY INFORMATION
Maple syrup	Adds flavor
Melon	Cantaloupe, honeydew, or watermelon
Milk	Nonfat, 1 percent, 2 percent, soy, almond, or rice
Miso	Adds flavor
Mushrooms	All varieties
Oatmeal	Absorbs acidity; make sure it's labeled gluten-free if you are gluten intolerant
Olive oil	1 to 2 tablespoons daily
Olives	Low acid
Pasta	With low-acid sauce—avoid if gluten sensitive
Pear	Ripe only, four or fewer per week—avoid if sensitive to FODMAPs
Popcorn	Air-popped only; no butter
Poultry	Skinless, not fried
Poultry broth or stock	Homemade is best
Rice	All types
Sea salt	This is not a low-sodium diet; however, if you have a history of hypertension, reduce the salt
Soy sauce	Great way to add flavor; choose gluten-free if needed
Sugar	Moderate amounts of brown or white sugar add flavor
Tofu	Excellent protein source for vegetarian meals
Vegetables, cruciferous	Broccoli, broccolini, broccoli rabe, cabbage, cauliflower
Vegetables, green	All, except for cucumbers (for some people) and green bell peppers
Vegetables, other	All unless otherwise noted
Vegetables, root (tubers)	Carrots, potatoes, rutabaga, sweet potato, turnips, etc.—noted exception: no onions
Yogurt	Low-fat, plain, nonfat, Greek-style—avoid if sensitive to FODMAPs

Culinary Creativity for GERD-Friendly Comfort Foods

Giving up your favorite foods can be difficult, even in pursuit of better health or fewer symptoms. However, as someone who has made this shift, I can assure you it is entirely worthwhile. Once your symptoms minimize or disappear, it's easy to look back and see the effort was worth it.

Standing here, looking ahead to drastic dietary changes, might feel vast, unwieldly, and difficult. I get it. However, learning tricks to make your new foods taste more like the old foods you love can help you feel like you're not sacrificing nearly as much on your journey to health.

Purée Root Vegetables with Broth

One of my all-time favorite comfort foods was rich, buttery mashed potatoes. Since butter is so limited on this type of diet, however, I needed a new way to get all the flavor and satisfaction without the buttery fat. You can purée any root veggie (depending on the amount) with a few tablespoons to $1/2$ cup of broth. The broth adds flavor and puréeing gives you the creaminess you long for in those mashed potatoes. When you're ready to eat, add just a teaspoon of butter to give you the flavor without all the fat.

Don't Skip the Salt

Even adding a pinch of salt brings out foods' natural flavors. Without salt, flavors fall flat. You don't need much, but you do need to salt your foods a little.

Nonfat Dairy Adds Creaminess

You can add creaminess to soups and other dishes with nonfat dairy products such as plain nonfat yogurt or fat-free sour cream. Stir in a few tablespoons to add richness and texture to your dishes.

Make Gravies, Thick Soups, & Sauces with Arrowroot, Cornstarch, or Puréed Root Vegetables

If you absolutely must have gravy on your meat and taters, there's a low-fat way to do it. Traditional gravy starts with a roux—a mix of fat and flour. Since you want to minimize fat, there are two tricks you can use to make a great gravy or sauce:

- Mix 3 tablespoons of arrowroot powder or cornstarch into 3 tablespoons of water. Whisk this slurry into hot broth and season appropriately.

- Purée cooked root vegetables (which are very starchy), such as carrots or potatoes, with hot broth and seasonings to make a thick soup base, gravy, or sauce.

Use the Proper Reflux-Friendly Cooking Method

Broiling, grilling, steaming, microwaving, dry sautéing, microwaving, and baking are all low-fat cooking methods that add plenty of flavor but allow you to avoid fat.

Cook with Juices or Broths Instead of Fats & Oils

This is a great stir-frying tip. Add just a teaspoon of oil and, as you need moisture for the cooking process, add broth or juice instead, a tablespoon at a time to keep your cooking low in fat.

Eat Acidic Foods with Alkaline Foods

One of the best ways to neutralize the acidity in foods you eat is to include other foods in your meal that are very alkaline. Grains, potatoes, and root veggies (except onions) are starchy, alkaline, and can soak up excess acid.

Don't Be Afraid of Herbs & Spices

Jazz up the flavors of all your foods with plenty of dried or fresh herbs and spices. With the exceptions of garlic, onions, chiles, and mint, anything goes as far as adding herbs and spices to your dishes. Experiment with making your own spice blends, and try mixing traditionally considered "sweet" spices (such as allspice, cinnamon, ginger, or nutmeg) into savory dishes. Likewise, try mixing traditionally savory herbs (such as thyme or rosemary) with sweet flavors like fruit. You just may discover a new flavor combination you adore.

Substitute Nut Milk or Rice Milk for Dairy If You Are Sensitive

If you're allergic to or have difficulty tolerating dairy, having a good substitution in your back pocket can help you feel like you're sacrificing less. Unsweetened rice milk, almond milk, or hemp milk are all great substitutions for dairy. Taste test and see which you prefer.

Bread & Bake, Don't Fry

You can approximate the flavor of your favorite fried foods by coating them with seasoned bread crumbs and baking to a crisp golden brown. It won't be as fatty, but it will still be flavorful.

Kitchen Equipment & Pantry List

As promised, you won't need any super-fancy or expensive equipment for these recipes, nor will you need exotic or expensive pantry items. I've designed them to be accessible and affordable.

Essential Equipment

Chances are, you probably already have most of this equipment in your kitchen. I recently furnished my college-age son's first apartment kitchen, and he could make these recipes from the simple equipment I bought him. (Okay—I donated my old stuff and bought new stuff for me, but you get the idea.) Here's what you'll need.

KNIVES

In my opinion, good-quality knives are the most important item you can have in your kitchen. You'll need one chef-style knife that you keep very sharp, as well as a paring knife, also very sharp.

CUTTING BOARD

You'll need two cutting boards—one for meat and one for everything else. It may be helpful to have them made of different materials so you know which is for which. The meat cutting board needs to be one you can easily sanitize with bleach or in the dishwasher.

MIXING BOWLS

You'll need three mixing bowls—small, medium, and large. They can be any material.

POTS & PANS

You'll need a basic assortment of pots and pans, including 8-, 10-, and 12-inch nonstick sauté pans or skillets, a large soup pot, and one or two medium saucepans. You'll also need a nonstick rimmed baking sheet, a rack for the baking sheet, a regular (6-muffin) muffin tin, and a mini (24-muffin) muffin tin (both preferably nonstick).

PARCHMENT PAPER

I'm a huge fan of parchment paper for baking because you can use it to line baking sheets and minimize sticking and cleanup. It also allows you to bake without greasing a pan.

BLENDER

A blender is great for making smoothies and purées. You can also use a food processor (if you have one) for this purpose.

INDOOR GRILL OR GRILL PAN

An indoor grill like a George Foreman grill or a stove top grill pan is a great piece of equipment when preparing meals for this diet. Grilling is one of the healthiest, low-fat ways to cook proteins. I love my George Foreman grill and use it a few times a week. It drains away the fat as it cooks the food.

RAMEKINS

Ramekins are your friend when portion control is of utmost importance. Find a good set of ovenproof 6- to 8-ounce ramekins. They allow you to bake individual portions, which cook more quickly and help you control how much you eat.

UTENSILS

You'll need one or two wooden spoons, heat-proof rubber spatulas, and silicone spatulas, as well as measuring cups (liquid and dry goods), and measuring spoons. You'll need a can opener and a box grater (the kind with different-size holes). You'll also need a vegetable peeler. If you're feeling super fancy, a rasp-style grater is also nice to have.

GERD-FRIENDLY INGREDIENT SUBSTITUTIONS

REMOVE	REPLACE
Barbecue sauce	Dijon mustard, fish sauce, liquid smoke, soy sauce
Broth, purchased	Broth, homemade
Cayenne pepper	Cumin
Chili powder	Cumin, coriander
Full-fat mayonnaise	Fat-free mayonnaise or nonfat Greek-style yogurt
Garlic powder, garlic salt	Basil, cumin, Dijon mustard, Italian seasoning
Ketchup	Anchovy fillets or paste, fish sauce, soy sauce, toasted sesame oil
Lemon juice, lime juice, orange juice	Lemon zest, lime zest, orange zest
MSG	Fish sauce, sea salt, soy sauce
Onion powder	Cumin, coriander, ginger, sea salt
Paprika	Cumin
Pepper	Cumin, Italian seasoning, oregano, thyme
Salad dressing	Salad dressing made with nonfat Greek-style yogurt, low-fat milk, or nut milks and herbs
Shortening/butter	Extra-virgin olive oil, nonstick cooking spray
Tomatoes, canned	Anchovy paste, Dijon mustard, fish sauce, soy sauce
Tuna, oil-packed	Tuna, water-packed

Pantry Staples

A well-stocked pantry makes it easy to pull out what you need to make meals. In your pantry, you'll need the following:

HERBS & SPICES

Get an assortment, including these:

- Allspice
- Black pepper, to be used sparingly
- Cinnamon, ground
- Cloves
- Dried oregano
- Dried rosemary
- Dried tarragon
- Dried thyme
- Ginger, fresh and ground
- Italian seasoning
- Nutmeg, ground
- Sea salt

OLIVE OIL

Get the best olive oil you can afford. My favorite is California Olive Ranch olive oil, which is a pure extra-virgin olive oil that comes in a variety of flavor levels (from deep and rich to light) based on your preference. Whichever oil you buy, make sure it is 100 percent olive oil—in the last few years, even mainstream brands have subtly blended other oils into their bottles, but they don't necessarily highlight it on the labels. Always read labels carefully.

DRIED GOODS

You'll also need a supply of dried goods, including these:

- Brown rice
- Cornstarch or arrowroot powder
- Flour, all-purpose, whole-wheat, and gluten-free
- Pasta (spaghetti, macaroni, orzo, etc.)
- Steel cut oats
- Sugar, brown and white

CANNED & BOTTLED ITEMS

For canned goods, stock the following:

- Beans, black and kidney
- Corn
- Honey
- Lentils
- Maple syrup, pure

CONDIMENTS

Flavorful condiments make foods more enjoyable. Consider keeping the following on hand:

- Dijon mustard
- Fat-free mayonnaise
- Fish sauce
- Soy sauce (choose gluten-free if you're sensitive)

RECIPE LABELS

As previously mentioned, the recipes in the following chapters include labels to help you determine which fits best for your unique needs.

- ALKALINE foods are okay for people in the strictest phases of the diet, and they don't have a pH lower than 5.

- GLUTEN-FREE foods are safe for people with celiac disease and non-celiac gluten sensitivity, as well as for those who wish to avoid gluten in their diets for other reasons.

- LOW-CARB RECIPES have 10 or fewer net grams (total carbs minus fiber) of carbs per serving.

- LOW-FODMAP recipes won't irritate IBS or IBD, and will help eliminate gassiness in people who process this type of carbohydrate poorly.

- PALEO recipes don't contain processed foods, industrial seed oils, sugars, legumes, or grains.

- VEGAN recipes don't contain any animal products, including honey.

- VEGETARIAN recipes don't contain any animal products except dairy, eggs, and honey.

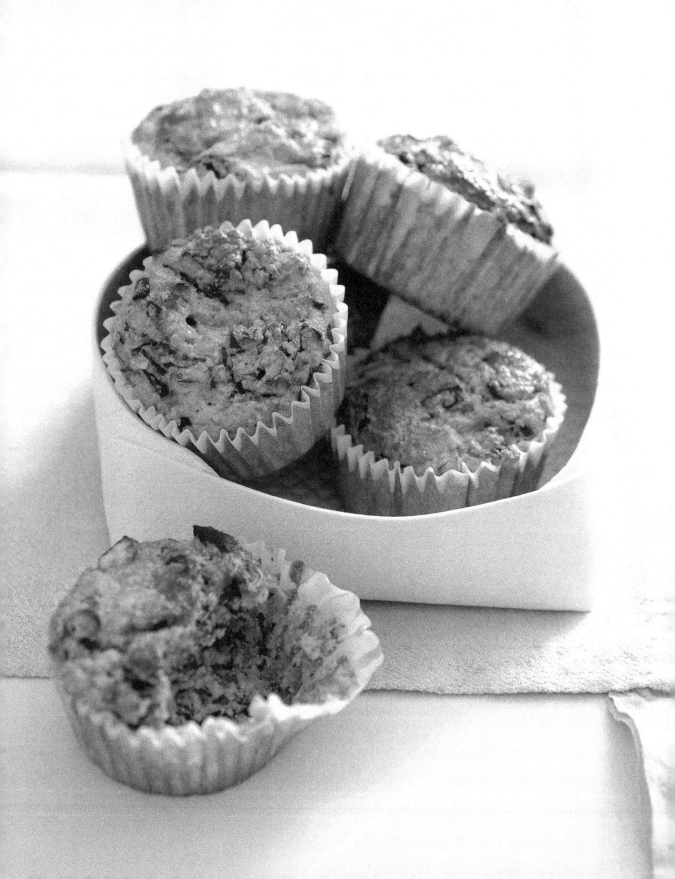

TWO

Smoothies & Breakfast

Zucchini-Bran Mini Muffins

ALKALINE   VEGETARIAN

Makes 24 muffins
Prep: 15 minutes
Cook: 15 minutes

These moist, rich muffins are a great way to use up that late-summer bounty of zucchini. Bran adds plenty of fiber and the muffins are lightly spiced, making for a slightly sweet breakfast. These freeze well—they last up to 12 months tightly sealed in a zip-top bag.

¾ cup all-purpose flour
1 teaspoon baking powder
1 teaspoon grated orange zest
½ teaspoon baking soda
½ teaspoon ground cinnamon
Pinch ground nutmeg
Pinch sea salt
½ cup sugar
3 tablespoons plus 1 teaspoon
    vegetable oil
1 egg
¾ cup grated zucchini
¼ cup wheat bran

1. Preheat the oven to 350°F.

2. Line a 24-cup mini muffin tin with mini cupcake liners.

3. In a medium bowl, mix the flour, baking powder, orange zest, baking soda, cinnamon, nutmeg, and salt.

4. In a small bowl, whisk together the sugar, oil, and egg. Add the wet ingredients to the dry ingredients and stir to combine. Do not overmix (see the tip).

5. Fold in the zucchini and the bran. Spoon batter into the prepared muffin cups, filling them three-fourths full.

6. Bake for 14 to 15 minutes until a toothpick inserted in the center of a muffin comes out clean.

tip   When stirring together the wet and dry ingredients, it's important to mix just until the batter comes together. There will be streaks of flour remaining in the mix. This keeps the crumb of the muffin tender.

PER SERVING (2 mini muffins) Calories: 113; Total Fat: 4g; Saturated Fat: <1g; Cholesterol: 14mg; Carbohydrates: 17g; Fiber: 1g; Protein: 2g; Sodium: 78mg

Ginger-Banana Smoothie

ALKALINE **GLUTEN-FREE** LOW-FODMAP PALEO VEGAN

Serves 2
Prep: 5 minutes

You can't get a much quicker or easier breakfast than a smoothie. Bananas have a pH of about 5, which means they are slightly acidic. However, they are also very starchy, so the starch absorbs the acidity and render bananas unlikely to cause heartburn.

2 cups unsweetened almond milk
1 banana
1 packet stevia
½ teaspoon grated fresh ginger
1 cup crushed ice

In a blender, combine the almond milk, banana, stevia, ginger, and ice. Blend until smooth.

tip If you are among the very small segment of the population who has acid reflux issues with bananas (like I did when I was pregnant), replace it with 2 cups cubed honeydew melon or cantaloupe.

PER SERVING (1½ cups) Calories: 158; Total Fat: 4g; Saturated Fat: 0g; Cholesterol: 0mg; Carbohydrates: 33g; Fiber: 3g; Protein: 2g; Sodium: 182mg

Pumpkin Pie Smoothie

ALKALINE **GLUTEN-FREE** **LOW-CARB** LOW-FODMAP PALEO VEGAN

Serves 2
Prep: 5 minutes

Pumpkin spice lovers, rejoice. While a pumpkin spice latte might cause a flare-up of your acid reflux, this flavorful smoothie allows you to get your pumpkin spice fix without regretting it later. Pumpkin is also rich in vitamin A and antioxidants, so it's a super-healthy way to start your day.

2 cups unsweetened almond milk
1½ cups canned pumpkin purée
¼ teaspoon grated fresh ginger
¼ teaspoon ground nutmeg
¼ teaspoon ground cinnamon
1 packet stevia
1 cup crushed ice

In a blender, combine the almond milk, pumpkin purée, ginger, nutmeg, cinnamon, stevia, and ice. Blend until smooth.

tip If you are allergic to tree nuts, replace the almond milk with an equal amount of rice milk.

PER SERVING (1½ cups) Calories: 169; Total Fat: 4g; Saturated Fat: <1g; Cholesterol: 0mg; Carbohydrates: 17g; Fiber: 7g; Protein: 3g; Sodium: 190mg

Maple–Brown Sugar Quick Grits

ALKALINE **GLUTEN-FREE** VEGAN

Serves 2
Prep: 5 minutes
Cook: 7 minutes

This hot and hearty breakfast is extremely satisfying. The slight earthiness of the corn combines beautifully with rich maple syrup and sweet brown sugar for a stick-to-your-ribs meal that tastes delicious. Be sure you purchase instant grits to keep your cooking time short.

1½ cups unsweetened almond milk
2 tablespoons pure maple syrup
1 tablespoon packed brown sugar
½ teaspoon ground cinnamon
Pinch sea salt
½ cup quick-cooking grits

1. In a small pot over high heat, bring the almond milk, maple syrup, brown sugar, cinnamon, and salt to a boil, stirring constantly. Reduce the heat to medium-high.

2. Stir in the grits. Cook for about 5 minutes, stirring constantly until the grits thicken.

tip If you can't find quick cooking grits, you can use wheat farina—just know that it is not gluten-free. For ½ cup, you'll need 2½ cups almond milk.

PER SERVING (1 cup) Calories: 130; Total Fat: 3g; Saturated Fat: 0g; Cholesterol: 0mg; Carbohydrates: 26g; Fiber: 2g; Protein: 1g; Sodium: 194mg

Oatmeal *with* Ginger *and* Dried Apples

GLUTEN-FREE VEGAN

Serves 2
Prep: 5 minutes
Cook: 5 minutes

If you are sensitive to gluten, it's important to note that some oats are processed in facilities that also process wheat products, so they may not be gluten-free. Look for oats that are certified gluten-free to ensure you don't accidentally get gluten contamination, which can set your efforts back. Many brands, such as Bob's Red Mill, offer specifically gluten-free oats.

2 cups unsweetened almond milk
2 tablespoons packed brown sugar (optional)
½ teaspoon grated fresh ginger
Pinch sea salt
1 cup rolled oats
¼ cup dried apples

1. In a small pot over high heat, bring the almond milk, brown sugar (if using), ginger, and salt to a boil. Reduce the heat to medium-high.

2. Stir in the oats. Cook for about 3 minutes, stirring constantly until the oats are soft.

3. Stir in the dried apples.

tip Dried apples may be too acidic for some people, although the starch in the oatmeal will help soak up the acid from the apples. If you are someone who finds that apples aggravate your acid reflux, stir in 1 tablespoon chopped almonds instead.

PER SERVING (1½ cups) Calories: 245;
Total Fat: 6g; Saturated Fat: <1g; Cholesterol: 0mg;
Carbohydrates: 43g; Fiber: 6g; Protein: 7g;
Sodium: 119mg

Cinnamon Granola

ALKALINE **GLUTEN-FREE** VEGAN

Serves 6
Prep: 5 minutes
Cook: 25 minutes

If you like a good, crunchy, low-fat breakfast cereal, you'll love this easy homemade granola. It takes about 25 minutes in the oven, but then you can store it in a tightly sealed container for a few weeks and have an easy breakfast on the go. Top it with skim milk, almond milk, or rice milk and some sliced banana for a tasty breakfast (or snack).

4 cups gluten-free rolled oats
½ cup water
½ cup pure maple syrup
¼ cup chopped almonds
1 teaspoon ground cinnamon

1. Preheat the oven to 300°F.

2. Line two baking sheets with parchment paper.

3. In a large bowl, combine the oats, water, maple syrup, almonds, and cinnamon. Mix well. Spread the granola in even layers on the prepared sheets.

4. Bake for about 25 minutes, stirring every 10 minutes, until golden.

tip Add ½ cup dried apples (if you tolerate them well) to the mixture before baking for extra flavor.

PER SERVING (1 cup) Calories: 316; Total Fat: 6g; Saturated Fat: <1g; Cholesterol: 0mg; Carbohydrates: 61g; Fiber: 6g; Protein: 8g; Sodium: 5mg

Mini Lemon-Cinnamon Muffins

ALKALINE VEGETARIAN

Serves 12
Prep: 10 minutes
Cook: 20 minutes, plus cooling

These freeze well, so they are perfect to make ahead for meals and snacks on those days when you simply don't have the time or energy to cook. Even though these muffins have lemon flavoring, it's not from the acidic lemon juice. Instead, it uses just a bit of lemon zest, which packs tremendous flavor from the citrus oils with very little acidity. You can also try orange zest or lime zest to make different flavors of tasty muffins.

¾ cup all-purpose flour
¾ cup whole-wheat flour
1 cup sugar, divided
2 teaspoons baking powder
Zest of 1 lemon
¼ teaspoon sea salt
2 tablespoons canola oil
2 tablespoons nonfat plain Greek-style yogurt
1 egg, beaten
½ cup unsweetened almond milk
½ teaspoon alcohol-free vanilla extract
1 teaspoon ground cinnamon
¼ cup unsalted butter, melted, divided

1. Preheat the oven to 400°F.

2. Line a 24-cup mini muffin tin with mini cupcake liners.

3. In a medium bowl, whisk together the flours, ¾ cup sugar, baking powder, lemon zest, and salt.

4. In another medium bowl, whisk together the oil, yogurt, egg, almond milk, and vanilla.

5. Add the wet ingredients to the dry ingredients and mix until just blended. There may be some streaks of flour remaining.

6. Fill each muffin cup one-half to three-fourths full with batter.

7. Bake for 15 to 20 minutes until the muffins are set and lightly browned on top. Transfer to a wire rack to cool.

8. In a small bowl, mix the remaining ¼ cup sugar and the cinnamon.

9. Brush each cooled muffin with ½ teaspoon the butter. Sprinkle with the cinnamon sugar.

tip If you can't find alcohol-free vanilla extract, try Simply Organic nonalcoholic Madagascar vanilla flavoring. It's available online and in most grocery stores. The very small amount used in recipes, particularly starchy recipes like this, is unlikely to aggravate GERD. However, you'll need to test yourself for tolerance to see if you need to purchase the alcohol-free vanilla or if you can use regular vanilla.

PER SERVING (2 mini muffins) Calories: 206; Total Fat: 9g; Saturated Fat: 5g; Cholesterol: 24mg; Carbohydrates: 30g; Fiber: <1g; Protein: 3g; Sodium: 76mg

Silver Dollar Pancakes with Brown Sugar Peaches

VEGAN

Serves 6
Prep: 15 minutes
Cook: 10 minutes

If you make tiny (silver dollar-size) pancakes, it's easy to keep your portions small so you don't overeat and aggravate your GERD. The topping uses canned peaches because they are less acidic than fresh. If you tolerate fresh peaches well, you can use those instead.

FOR THE PANCAKES

1¼ cups whole-wheat flour
2 teaspoons baking powder
Pinch sea salt
1¼ cups unsweetened almond milk
½ teaspoon alcohol-free vanilla extract
Nonstick cooking spray

FOR THE PEACHES

1 (14-ounce) can peaches in juice, drained
¼ cup packed brown sugar
½ teaspoon ground ginger

TO MAKE THE PANCAKES

1. In a medium bowl, whisk together the flour, baking powder, and salt.

2. In a small bowl or in a liquid measuring cup, stir together the almond milk and vanilla.

3. Add the wet ingredients to the dry ingredients and stir until just combined.

4. Heat a nonstick griddle or sauté pan over medium-high heat. Spray it with nonstick cooking spray.

5. Working in 2-tablespoon measures, pour the pancakes onto the griddle. Cook the pancakes for about 3 minutes, until bubbles form on top. Flip and cook for 3 minutes more.

TO MAKE THE PEACHES

1. In a blender, purée the peaches for about 1 minute until smooth.

2. In a small saucepan over medium heat, stir together the peaches, brown sugar, and ginger.

3. Simmer for 3 minutes, stirring constantly. Serve over the pancakes.

tip If peaches are a bit acidic for you, use pure maple syrup to top your pancakes. It's fat-free, delicious, and traditional.

PER SERVING (2 pancakes with ¼ cup topping)
Calories: 267; Total Fat: 2g; Saturated Fat: 0g; Cholesterol: 0mg; Carbohydrates: 59g; Fiber: 6g; Protein: 6g; Sodium: 38mg

Spinach Frittata

ALKALINE **LOW-CARB** LOW-FODMAP PALEO VEGETARIAN

Serves 4
Prep: 10 minutes
Cook: 10 minutes

Egg dishes freeze well, which makes them great for doubling a recipe, cutting it into pieces, and freezing in a zip-top bag for quick meals later. I do this with frittatas and egg casseroles all the time, which helps me stay on track when I'm just too busy to cook. Reheat them in the microwave for about two minutes on high (frozen) or one minute on high (thawed).

2 teaspoons extra-virgin olive oil
1½ cups fresh baby spinach
1 teaspoon grated orange zest
½ teaspoon sea salt
¼ teaspoon ground nutmeg
6 eggs, beaten
2 tablespoons water

1. Preheat the broiler to high.

2. In a 10- to 12-inch ovenproof nonstick skillet over medium-high heat, heat the olive oil until it shimmers.

3. Add the spinach, orange zest, salt, and nutmeg. Cook for about 1 minute, stirring occasionally until the spinach is wilted. Reduce the heat to medium. Spread the spinach in an even layer over the bottom of the skillet.

4. In a small bowl, whisk together the eggs and water. Gently add the eggs to the skillet and stir lightly to distribute evenly with the spinach. Cook for about 3 minutes, until the eggs are set around the edges.

5. Transfer the pan to the broiler. Broil for 3 to 4 minutes until the eggs are browned and puffy on top. Cut into wedges and serve.

tip Before transferring the pan to the broiler, gently sprinkle ¼ cup grated Cheddar cheese (if you tolerate it well) over the top in an even layer.

PER SERVING (¼ frittata) Calories: 118; Total Fat: 9g; Saturated Fat: 2g; Cholesterol: 246mg; Carbohydrates: 1g; Fiber: <1g; Protein: 9g; Sodium: 336mg

Cheesy Scrambled Eggs

LOW-CARB LOW-FODMAP VEGETARIAN

Serves 2
Prep: 5 minutes
Cook: 7 minutes

Pump up your scrambled eggs with lots of flavor using spices and cheese. You can adjust the herbs and spices to meet your own taste preferences, or even just sprinkle in a little salt for a tasty high-protein breakfast.

Nonstick cooking spray
4 eggs
¼ teaspoon sea salt
¼ teaspoon ground cumin
2 tablespoons chopped fresh cilantro
¼ cup grated Monterey Jack cheese

1. Spray a 10-inch nonstick sauté pan or skillet with nonstick cooking spray and place it over medium heat.

2. In a small bowl, whisk together the eggs, salt, and cumin. Pour the eggs into the heated pan and cook for about 5 minutes, stirring frequently until set.

3. Stir in the cilantro and cheese. Cook for 1 to 2 minutes more, stirring until the cheese melts.

tip Make huevos rancheros by stirring in one-half of a tomato (if you tolerate it well), chopped, and ¼ cup black beans with the cheese. Cook for a few minutes until the beans heat through.

PER SERVING (about ½ cup) Calories: 180; Total Fat: 13g; Saturated Fat: 5g; Cholesterol: 340mg; Carbohydrates: <1g; Fiber: 0g; Protein: 15g; Sodium: 434mg

Mushroom *and* Turkey Bacon Omelet

ALKALINE **LOW-CARB** PALEO

Serves 2
Prep: 10 minutes
Cook: 20 minutes

If it's an omelet you crave, you're in luck. This easy omelet serves two and makes for a protein-filled, satisfying breakfast that will get your day off to a great start. If omelet preparation (rolling the eggs) seems a bit of a hassle, no worries. Just scramble the eggs around the mushrooms and bacon. It won't look as pretty, but it will be just as delicious.

2 teaspoons extra-virgin olive oil
4 turkey bacon slices, cut into pieces
1 cup sliced mushrooms
4 eggs, beaten
1 tablespoon water
¼ teaspoon sea salt

tip Before rolling the omelet, sprinkle 2 tablespoons grated Parmesan cheese (if you tolerate it well) over the top. Allow it to melt slightly, for about 1 minute, before rolling.

1. In an 8- or 10-inch nonstick sauté pan or skillet over medium-high heat, heat the olive oil until it shimmers.

2. Add the turkey bacon and cook for about 5 minutes, stirring occasionally until browned.

3. Add the mushrooms. Cook for about 5 minutes, stirring occasionally until soft.

4. In a small bowl, whisk together the eggs, water, and salt.

5. Reduce the heat under the skillet to medium. Pour the eggs over the cooked mushrooms and bacon. Cook the eggs for about 4 minutes or until set around the edges.

6. With a rubber spatula, carefully pull the solidified mixture away from the edges and tilt the pan to allow the uncooked eggs to run underneath. Continue cooking for about 3 minutes more until the eggs are solidified around the edges again.

7. With a spatula, carefully lift one edge of the eggs and roll the omelet. It may help to tilt the pan at an angle. Cook 1 minute more.

PER SERVING (½ omelet) Calories: 213;
Total Fat: 15g; Saturated Fat: 3g; Cholesterol: 347mg;
Carbohydrates: 2g; Fiber: 0g; Protein: 18g;
Sodium: 599mg

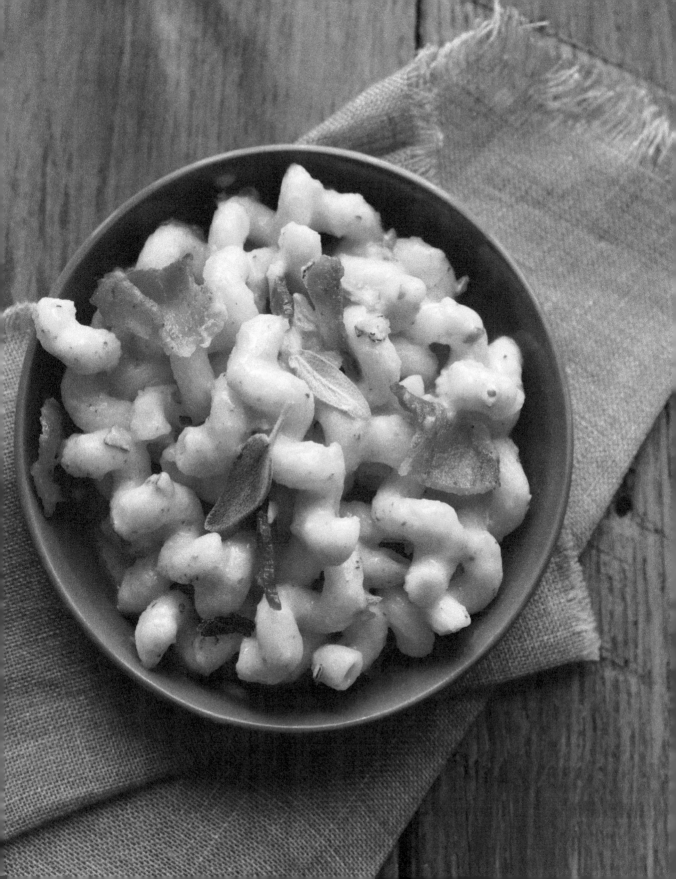

THREE

Appetizers & Sides

Cinnamon Apple "Fries"

GLUTEN-FREE PALEO VEGAN

Serves 4
Prep: 10 minutes
Cook: 12 minutes

Quick, easy, and delicious, these apple "fries" are just what you need for a mid-morning snack or something to enjoy on the go. While they are tastiest when hot, you can also serve them cold. They are also the ultimate in versatility. You can replace the cinnamon with your favorite sweet spice (nutmeg and ginger are both nice), or even add just a savory hint by using chopped rosemary or thyme. Yum!

2 red apples, peeled, cored, and cut
    into wedges
1 tablespoon melted coconut oil
1 tablespoon pure maple syrup
1 teaspoon ground cinnamon
Pinch sea salt

1. Preheat the oven to 375°F.

2. Line a baking sheet with parchment paper.

3. In a large bowl, toss together the apples, coconut oil, maple syrup, cinnamon, and salt until evenly coated. Spread the apples in a single layer on the prepared sheet.

4. Bake for about 12 minutes until the apples are browned.

tip Need something a little more alkaline? Use one sweet potato or half a butternut squash instead of the apples. You'll need to increase the baking time by about 10 minutes, but both have fantastic flavor with the sweet spices.

PER SERVING (¼ cup) Calories: 98; Total Fat: 2g; Saturated Fat: 2g; Cholesterol: 8mg; Carbohydrates: 19g; Fiber: 3g; Protein: <1g; Sodium: 61mg

Bacon-Wrapped Melon

ALKALINE **GLUTEN-FREE** **LOW-CARB** LOW-FODMAP PALEO

Serves 4
Prep: 10 minutes

When you can combine sweet and salty in one easy-to-make, no-cook food, you have something to celebrate. While the recipe calls for cantaloupe, honeydew melon works equally well. Use paper-thin slices of Canadian bacon, which is low in fat and delicious with the melon.

½ cantaloupe, rind removed and seeded, cut into 8 wedges
8 very thin Canadian bacon slices

Wrap each melon wedge with 1 piece of Canadian bacon and secure with a toothpick.

tip Looking to pump up the sweet and savory? Sprinkle the melon wedges with about 1 teaspoon chopped fresh thyme, and drizzle the wrapped slices with 2 tablespoons honey.

PER SERVING (2 pieces) Calories: 28; Total Fat: 1g; Saturated Fat: 0g; Cholesterol: 7mg; Carbohydrates: 2g; Fiber: 0g; Protein: 3g; Sodium: 302mg

Honeyed Mini Corn Muffins

Serves 12
Prep: 5 minutes
Cook: 15 minutes

Lightly sweet mini corn muffins make a delicious side dish for soups or stews, or they're great as a snack on their own. If you're vegan, replace the honey in this recipe with an equal amount of pure maple syrup, which adds a warm, sweet flavor.

1¾ cups cornmeal

¾ cup all-purpose flour

1 tablespoon baking powder

1 teaspoon baking soda

¼ teaspoon sea salt

1½ cups unsweetened almond milk

¼ cup honey

2 eggs, beaten

2 tablespoons canola oil

2 tablespoons nonfat plain
    Greek-style yogurt

1. Preheat the oven to 425°F.

2. Line a 24-cup mini muffin tin with mini cupcake liners.

3. In a medium bowl, whisk the cornmeal, flour, baking powder, baking soda, and salt together.

4. In another medium bowl, whisk together the almond milk, honey, eggs, oil, and yogurt.

5. Add the wet ingredients to the dry ingredients and mix until just combined. Fill each muffin cup half to three-fourths full.

6. Bake for about 15 minutes, or until a toothpick inserted in the center comes out clean.

tip Add the zest of 1 orange to the wet ingredients to add a citrusy flavor boost.

PER SERVING (2 mini muffins) Calories: 217; Total Fat: 11g; Saturated Fat: 7g; Cholesterol: 27mg; Carbohydrates: 28g; Fiber: 2g; Protein: 4g; Sodium: 167mg

Buttermilk Biscuits

VEGETARIAN

Serves 8
Prep: 15 minutes
Cook: 15 minutes

While buttermilk is slightly acidic, the starch in the flour absorbs it well. If you find you are still a bit sensitive to buttermilk, replace it with any low-fat nondairy milk, like almond milk. You'll sacrifice a bit of flavor, but you can add it back by adding one teaspoon grated lemon zest.

¾ cup all-purpose flour

¾ cup whole-wheat flour

1 teaspoon baking soda

½ teaspoon sea salt

2 tablespoons cold unsalted butter, cut into small pieces

½ cup nonfat plain Greek-style yogurt

¼ cup low-fat buttermilk

2 tablespoons honey

1. Preheat the oven to 425°F.

2. Line a baking sheet with parchment paper.

3. In a medium bowl, whisk together the flours, baking soda, and salt.

4. Using two knives or a pastry blender, cut in the butter until the mixture resembles coarse oatmeal.

5. Stir in the yogurt, buttermilk, and honey.

6. Drop the dough in 8 equal portions onto the prepared sheet. Shape them lightly into rounds.

7. Bake for 14 to 15 minutes until golden brown.

tip To make the biscuits very flaky, it is important that the butter is very cold. Cut it into small pieces and freeze it for 30 minutes to 1 hour before cooking for the flakiest biscuits.

PER SERVING (1 biscuit) Calories: 138; Total Fat: 3g; Saturated Fat: 2g; Cholesterol: 8mg; Carbohydrates: 24g; Fiber: <1g; Protein: 4g; Sodium: 317mg

Baked Tortilla Chips *with* Black Bean Dip

ALKALINE **GLUTEN-FREE** VEGAN

Serves 4
Prep: 10 minutes
Cook: 15 minutes

Who doesn't love chips and dip? With a flavorful (and super-quick) bean dip and homemade tortilla chips, you can snack to your heart's content—just remember to keep portions small.

4 corn tortillas, cut into 8 wedges each

1 teaspoon sea salt, divided

1 (14-ounce) can black beans, drained and rinsed

1 teaspoon ground cumin

½ teaspoon ground coriander

2 tablespoons chopped fresh cilantro

1. Preheat the oven to 350°F.

2. Line a baking sheet with parchment paper.

3. Spread the tortilla wedges in a single layer on the prepared sheet. Sprinkle with ¼ teaspoon of salt.

4. Bake for about 15 minutes.

5. Meanwhile, in a medium saucepan over medium-high heat, warm the black beans, cumin, coriander, and the remaining ¾ teaspoon of salt for 5 minutes, stirring occasionally.

6. Transfer the mixture to a blender or food processor and process until smooth. Stir in the cilantro and serve with the warm tortilla chips.

tip You can use an equal amount of your favorite canned beans here, such as kidney or pinto beans, which will give the dip a slightly different flavor and consistency.

PER SERVING (8 tortilla wedges with ¼ cup dip) Calories: 393; Total Fat: 2g; Saturated Fat: 0g; Cholesterol: 0mg; Carbohydrates: 73g; Fiber: 16g; Protein: 23g; Sodium: 485mg

Jicama *with* Low-Fat Ranch Dip

ALKALINE **GLUTEN-FREE** **LOW-CARB** VEGETARIAN

Serves 8
Prep: 10 minutes

Chips and dip is a pretty standard appetizer or snack, but traditional chips and dips are usually high in fat, which can cause acid reflux flare-ups. This version is tasty and low fat, substituting satisfying, crunchy jicama for fried potato chips. It also travels well, so it's perfect to take as an on-the-go snack or a party appetizer.

1 cup fat-free cottage cheese
1 cup fat-free sour cream
2 tablespoons chopped fresh dill
1 tablespoon chopped fresh thyme
1 teaspoon chopped fresh chives
1 teaspoon grated lemon zest
½ teaspoon sea salt
1 jicama, peeled and sliced

In a medium bowl, stir together the cottage cheese, sour cream, dill, thyme, chives, lemon zest, and salt. Serve with the sliced jicama for dipping.

tip You can find jicama with the root veggies in the produce section of the grocery store. If you can't find jicama (or don't like it), replace it with carrot sticks.

PER SERVING (½ cup sliced veggies with ¼ cup dip)
Calories: 90; Total Fat: <1g; Saturated Fat: 0g; Cholesterol: 5mg; Carbohydrates: 14g; Fiber: 4g; Protein: 6g; Sodium: 262mg

Baked Green Bean "Fries" *with* French Fry Sauce

ALKALINE **LOW-CARB**

Serves 4
Prep: 10 minutes
Cook: 15 minutes

Crave French fries? You're not alone. I love them, but they certainly don't love me. These green bean fries are a tasty substitute, and the dipping sauce is a flavorful accompaniment. These are great as a side dish, or they make a tasty snack.

Nonstick cooking spray
¾ cup bread crumbs
1 teaspoon dried thyme
½ teaspoon dried rosemary
½ teaspoon sea salt
¼ teaspoon ground cumin
2 eggs, beaten
1 teaspoon Dijon mustard
1 pound fresh green beans, trimmed
    and halved
1 cup French Fry Sauce (page 145)

1. Preheat the oven to 425°F.

2. Spray a baking sheet with nonstick cooking spray.

3. In a large bowl, mix the bread crumbs, thyme, rosemary, salt, and cumin.

4. In another large bowl, whisk the eggs and mustard together.

5. Add the green beans to the egg mixture and stir to coat.

6. Toss the coated beans with the bread crumbs to coat. Place them in a single layer on the prepared sheet.

7. Bake for about 12 minutes until golden brown. Flip and bake for 3 minutes more. Serve with the dipping sauce.

tip Sensitive to gluten? Gluten-free bread crumbs (homemade or purchased at your local health food store) put these fries within your reach. For a paleo version, replace the bread crumbs with almond meal. For a vegetarian version, serve without the French Fry Sauce.

PER SERVING (½ cup beans with ¼ cup sauce)
Calories: 100; Total Fat: 2g; Saturated Fat: <1g; Cholesterol: 43mg; Carbohydrates: 13g; Fiber: 3g; Protein: 8g; Sodium: 607mg

Baked Potato Chips

ALKALINE **GLUTEN-FREE** LOW-FODMAP VEGAN

Serves 4
Prep: 5 minutes
Cook: 25 minutes

If it's potato chips you love, don't worry—you can still have them. You just need to bake them instead of deep-frying them. The great thing about these chips is you can customize them by adding herbs and spices, or just enjoy them in their plain, slightly salty glory. Try them with any of the suggested dips in chapter 8 (starting on page 131).

Nonstick cooking spray

1 medium russet potato, cut into ¼-inch-thick slices

2 tablespoons extra-virgin olive oil

½ teaspoon sea salt

1. Preheat the oven to 400°F.

2. Spray a baking sheet with nonstick cooking spray.

3. In a large bowl, mix the potato slices, oil, and salt to coat. Spread the chips in a single layer on the prepared sheet.

4. Bake for about 25 minutes until crisp and brown.

tip Want to make it paleo? Replace the potato with a sweet potato—no need to peel.

PER SERVING (½ cup) Calories: 131; Total Fat: 7g; Saturated Fat: 1g; Cholesterol: 0mg; Carbohydrates: 16g; Fiber: 2g; Protein: 2g; Sodium: 237mg

Sweet Potato Oven "Fries"

ALKALINE **GLUTEN-FREE** **LOW-CARB** PALEO VEGAN

Serves 4
Prep: 5 minutes
Cook: 25 minutes

Crispy on the outside, fluffy on the inside, these oven "fries" are another tasty substitute for high-fat, deep-fried, acid reflux–causing French fries. Aren't you happy there are so many tasty alternatives? Of course, you can also make this recipe with regular potatoes if sweet potatoes aren't your thing. Try these with Curry Mayonnaise (page 146) for an extra kick.

Nonstick cooking spray
1 medium sweet potato, cut into
    ¼-inch-thick strips
2 tablespoons extra-virgin olive oil
½ teaspoon sea salt

1. Preheat the oven to 450°F.

2. Spray a baking sheet with nonstick cooking spray.

3. In a large bowl, mix the sweet potato strips, oil, and salt to coat. Spread the fries in a single layer on the prepared sheet.

4. Bake for about 25 minutes until crisp and brown.

tip This recipe is also delicious with butternut squash (½ squash), as well as peeled celery root (1 to 2 roots), which is perfect if you want to make it low-FODMAP (limit your serving to about ¼ cup of squash).

PER SERVING (½ cup) Calories: 101; Total Fat: 7g; Saturated Fat: 1g; Cholesterol: 0mg; Carbohydrates: 9g; Fiber: 2g; Protein: <1g; Sodium: 244mg

Roasted Parmesan Potatoes

ALKALINE **GLUTEN-FREE** LOW-FODMAP VEGETARIAN

Serves 4
Prep: 10 minutes
Cook: 20 minutes

Is there anything tastier as a side dish than roasted potatoes? I didn't think so! With a golden-brown exterior and lots of flavor from fresh rosemary and Parmesan cheese, these potatoes make a delicious accompaniment to poultry or fish.

Nonstick cooking spray
2 cups diced Yukon Gold potatoes (½-inch pieces)
2 tablespoons extra-virgin olive oil
½ teaspoon sea salt
1 tablespoon chopped fresh rosemary
2 tablespoons grated Parmesan cheese

1. Preheat the oven to 450°F.

2. Spray a baking sheet with nonstick cooking spray.

3. In a large bowl, mix the potatoes, oil, salt, and rosemary to coat. Place the potatoes in a single layer on the prepared sheet.

4. Bake for about 20 minutes until crisp and brown.

5. Toss with the Parmesan cheese before serving.

tip Want to make it vegan or don't tolerate cheese well? Replace the Parmesan cheese with 2 tablespoons nutritional yeast, which has a lovely cheesy flavor.

PER SERVING (½ cup) Calories: 113; Total Fat: 7g; Saturated Fat: 1g; Cholesterol: 0mg; Carbohydrates: 12g; Fiber: 1g; Protein: 1g; Sodium: 271mg

Maple-Thyme Roasted Carrots

ALKALINE **GLUTEN-FREE** PALEO VEGAN

Serves 4
Prep: 10 minutes
Cook: 20 minutes

When you roast root vegetables, they take on a savory, caramelized flavor that lights up your palate. These carrots are no exception. Sweet maple syrup and carrots are perfectly accented by fragrant, aromatic thyme, making this a delicious side dish for any meal.

Nonstick cooking spray
4 carrots, peeled and cut lengthwise
   into quarters
2 tablespoons extra-virgin olive oil
1 teaspoon grated orange zest
½ teaspoon sea salt
½ teaspoon dried thyme
2 tablespoons pure maple syrup

1. Preheat the oven to 400°F.

2. Spray a baking sheet with nonstick cooking spray.

3. In a large bowl, mix the carrots, oil, orange zest, salt, and thyme to coat. Spread the carrots in a single layer on the prepared sheet.

4. Bake for about 20 minutes, until the carrots are brown and roasted.

5. Toss with the maple syrup before serving.

tip This recipe also works well with other root vegetables, especially those that are slightly sweet, such as beets or parsnips.

PER SERVING (½ cup) Calories: 118;
Total Fat: 7g; Saturated Fat: 1g; Cholesterol: 0mg;
Carbohydrates: 15g; Fiber: 2g; Protein: <1g;
Sodium: 277mg

Mac 'n' Cheese

Serves 4
Prep: 15 minutes
Cook: 5 minutes

Eat like a kid again with this delicious mac 'n' cheese. It's easy to make and tastes of cheesy goodness that will take you right back to childhood—without all the excess fat to aggravate your acid reflux. This freezes well, so you can make it and save it in individual portions for ready-made meals.

3 cups (1 recipe) Low-Fat White Sauce (page 136)

2 ounces fat-free sharp Cheddar cheese, grated

6 ounces whole-wheat elbow macaroni, cooked according to package directions and drained

1 tablespoon melted unsalted butter

¼ cup bread crumbs

1. Preheat the broiler to high.

2. In a medium saucepan over medium heat, cook the white sauce and Cheddar cheese for 2 to 3 minutes, whisking constantly until the cheese melts.

3. Add the hot macaroni and toss to coat. Evenly divide among four (6-ounce) ramekins, or spread into a baking dish.

4. In a small bowl, mix the butter and bread crumbs. Sprinkle over the mac 'n' cheese.

5. Broil for 1 to 2 minutes until the bread crumbs are golden brown.

tip Add a bit of crunch and smokiness by chopping up grilled bacon slices to serve as a topping. Fresh herbs also make for an aromatic and colorful addition.

PER SERVING (1 ramekin) Calories: 258;
Total Fat: 5g; Saturated Fat: 2g; Cholesterol: 14mg;
Carbohydrates: 41g; Fiber: 4g; Protein: 12g;
Sodium: 343mg

Quick Rice Pilaf

ALKALINE **GLUTEN-FREE** VEGAN

Serves 4
Prep: 10 minutes
Cook: 11 minutes

Using precooked rice helps this recipe come together quickly. You can find cooked rice alongside regular rice at the grocery store or in the freezer section. You can also cook brown rice ahead of time and freeze in one-cup servings for convenience.

2 tablespoons extra-virgin olive oil
1 carrot, peeled and cut into ¼-inch dice
½ apple, peeled and cut into ¼-inch dice
¼ cup slivered almonds
1 teaspoon dried thyme
½ teaspoon sea salt
1 cup cooked brown rice
¼ cup Vegetable Broth (page 134)

1. In a large sauté pan or skillet over medium-high heat, heat the oil until it shimmers.

2. Add the carrot, apple, almonds, thyme, and salt. Cook for about 5 minutes, stirring occasionally until the apples and carrots are soft.

3. Stir in the rice and broth. Cook for 5 minutes more, stirring occasionally.

tip If apples are too acidic for you, leave them out of the recipe and add another carrot instead.

PER SERVING (¼ cup) Calories: 290;
Total Fat: 11g; Saturated Fat: 2g; Cholesterol: 0mg;
Carbohydrates: 43g; Fiber: 4g; Protein: 5g;
Sodium: 295mg

Mushroom *and* Pea Couscous

ALKALINE VEGAN

Serves 4
Prep: 10 minutes
Cook: 10 minutes
Rest: 10 minutes

Many people don't realize couscous is actually tiny bits of pasta. Therefore, it's not great for people with gluten or FODMAP sensitivities. However, if you don't have those sensitivities, this makes a delicious and quick side dish, and a tasty vegan meal.

1 tablespoon extra-virgin olive oil
1 cup sliced mushrooms
1 cup peas, fresh or frozen
1½ cups Vegetable Broth (page 134)
½ teaspoon dried thyme
¼ teaspoon sea salt
1 cup couscous

1. In a medium pot over medium-high heat, heat the oil until it shimmers.

2. Add the mushrooms and cook for 5 minutes, stirring occasionally.

3. Add the peas, broth, thyme, and salt. Bring to a boil.

4. Remove from the heat and stir in the couscous. Cover and let sit for 10 minutes. Fluff with a fork.

tip Want to make it gluten-free? Heat some cooked brown rice in the microwave. Omit the broth and couscous. Sauté the mushrooms and peas with the sea salt and thyme, and stir in the rice.

PER SERVING (¼ cup) Calories: 240; Total Fat: 5g; Saturated Fat: <1g; Cholesterol: 0mg; Carbohydrates: 40g; Fiber: 4g; Protein: 10g; Sodium: 410mg

Simple Sautéed Greens

ALKALINE **GLUTEN-FREE** **LOW-CARB** LOW-FODMAP PALEO VEGAN

Serves 4
Prep: 5 minutes
Cook: 10 minutes

If you dig greens, this versatile dish is perfect for you. You can use any greens you love—from collard greens to kale to spinach or any other tasty seasonally available greens like beet greens and mustard greens. You can also vary the herbs and spices for your personal taste. I am a huge fan of a little lemon zest with the greens, but you may like something else.

2 tablespoons extra-virgin olive oil
4 cups chopped kale, or other green of choice
2 tablespoons Vegetable Broth (page 134)
Zest of 1 lemon
½ teaspoon sea salt
Pinch ground nutmeg

1. In a 10- or 12-inch sauté pan or skillet over medium-high heat, heat the oil until it shimmers.

2. Add the kale, broth, and lemon zest. Cook for 5 to 10 minutes, stirring constantly until the kale is very soft.

3. Season with the salt and nutmeg. Serve immediately.

tip Sprinkle 2 tablespoons grated Parmesan cheese (if you tolerate it well) and 2 slices browned and crumbled turkey bacon over the top for a pop of flavor.

PER SERVING (¼ cup) Calories: 95; Total Fat: 7g; Saturated Fat: 1g; Cholesterol: 0mg; Carbohydrates: 7g; Fiber: 1g; Protein: 2g; Sodium: 287mg

Mixed Veggie Stir-Fry

ALKALINE **GLUTEN-FREE** **LOW-CARB** VEGAN

Serves 4
Prep: 5 minutes
Cook: 7 minutes

Love peas and carrots? Add flavor by stir-frying them with other veggies for a tasty vegetable medley. This is another dish that customizes easily, so add your low-acid favorites for a quick and easy side dish. Mix with rice for a great vegan entrée.

2 tablespoons extra-virgin olive oil
1 cup sliced mushrooms
1 cup peas, fresh or frozen
1 carrot, peeled and diced
1 cup broccoli florets
½ teaspoon ground ginger
2 tablespoons gluten-free soy sauce

1. In a 10- or 12-inch sauté pan or skillet over medium-high heat, heat the oil until it shimmers.

2. Add the mushrooms, peas, carrot, broccoli, and ginger. Cook for about 5 minutes, stirring frequently until the veggies are soft.

3. Stir in the soy sauce. Simmer for 1 minute more.

tip For a paleo version, replace the peas with 1 cup cauliflower florets.

PER SERVING (¼ cup) Calories: 110;
Total Fat: 7g; Saturated Fat: 1g; Cholesterol: 0mg;
Carbohydrates: 10g; Fiber: 3g; Protein: 3g;
Sodium: 499mg

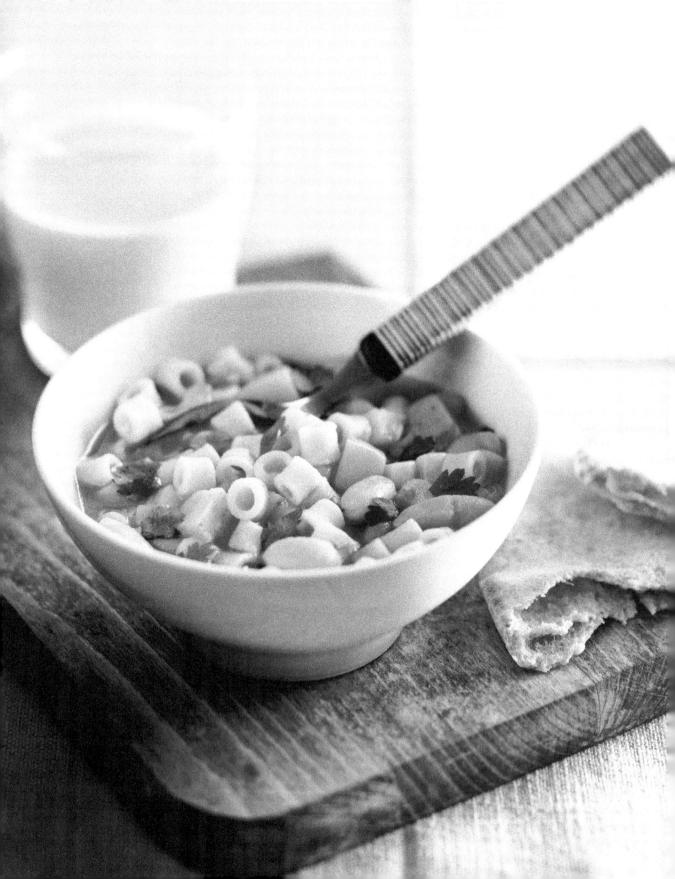

FOUR

Salads, Soups & Sandwiches

Ambrosia Salad

GLUTEN-FREE VEGETARIAN

Serves 6
Prep: 10 minutes
Chill: 15 minutes to 1 hour (see tip)

A mainstay at family gatherings and pot-lucks, the typical ambrosia salad is often an acid reflux trigger waiting to happen, with its high-acid fruits and fatty whipped cream. This version trims the fat and uses reflux-friendly fruits to give you all the creamy goodness of a typical ambrosia salad without the pain.

1 red apple, peeled, cored, and chopped

1 banana, peeled and chopped

½ cantaloupe, rind removed and seeded, cubed

½ cup nonfat plain Greek-style yogurt

1 tablespoon honey

1 teaspoon grated orange zest

1. In a large bowl, stir together the apple, banana, and cantaloupe.

2. In a small bowl, whisk together the yogurt, honey, and orange zest.

3. Gently toss the dressing with the fruit. Refrigerate for 1 hour before serving.

tip Freeze for 15 minutes if you need to serve this quickly.

PER SERVING (¼ cup) Calories: 66; Total Fat: <1g; Saturated Fat: 0g; Cholesterol: 1mg; Carbohydrates: 15g; Fiber: 2g; Protein: 2g; Sodium: 18mg

Creamy Coleslaw

ALKALINE **GLUTEN-FREE LOW-CARB** PALEO VEGETARIAN

Serves 6
Prep: 10 minutes

Sometimes, the only salad that will satisfy is a creamy coleslaw. Although it is alkaline, raw cabbage may trigger acid reflux in some people because it causes gas, which increases IAP. That's why this coleslaw uses grated carrots and jicama, which can mimic the crunchy, cool texture of cabbage with less chance of causing discomfort.

2 large carrots, peeled and grated or julienned
1 jicama, peeled and grated or julienned
¼ cup Creamy Avocado Coleslaw Dressing
    (page 147)

In a large bowl, toss the carrots and jicama with the dressing until coated.

tip If cabbage doesn't aggravate your GERD, try using 1½ cups shredded cabbage instead of the carrots and jicama. Or use other raw grated root vegetables, such as beets, to add a pop of color and a hint of sweetness. You can also julienne or finely chop the vegetables in this recipe if you don't have a grater (or prefer to show off your knife skills!).

PER SERVING (¼ cup) Calories: 62; Total Fat: 1g; Saturated Fat: 0g; Cholesterol: 0mg; Carbohydrates: 12g; Fiber: 6g; Protein: 1g; Sodium: 99mg

Carrot *and* Apple Salad

GLUTEN-FREE LOW-CARB VEGETARIAN

Serves 6
Prep: 10 minutes

Carrot and raisin salad has long been a popular side dish for family gatherings and potlucks, but raisins are just a bit acidic and may trigger acid reflux. This recipe uses red apple in place of the raisins, which mimics the sweetness in a traditional carrot and raisin salad without the acid reflux.

4 large carrots, peeled and grated
½ red apple, peeled, cored, and diced
¼ cup Greek Yogurt "Mayonnaise" (page 138)

In a large bowl, stir together the carrots, apple, and mayonnaise until the carrots and apples are coated.

tip While dried apples may be a bit acidic for some, if you don't have a problem with them, replace the fresh apple with ¼ cup dried apple pieces instead. This adds a more intense apple flavor and offers a texture similar to raisins.

PER SERVING (¼ cup) Calories: 35; Total Fat: <1g; Saturated Fat: 0g; Cholesterol: 0mg; Carbohydrates: 8g; Fiber: 1g; Protein: 1g; Sodium: 118mg

Potato Salad

ALKALINE **GLUTEN-FREE**

Serves 8
Prep: 10 minutes, plus cooling
Cook: 10 minutes

Potato salad doesn't have to trigger acid reflux. The trick is to eat small portions and minimize the amount of fat in it. In most cases, most of the fat in potato salad comes from mayonnaise, and a typical potato salad includes onions. This recipe avoids both of these known reflux triggers.

½ teaspoon sea salt

3 large potatoes, peeled and cut into
    ½-inch cubes

3 turkey bacon slices, cooked and crumbled

2 hardboiled eggs, peeled and chopped

1 celery stalk, finely chopped

½ cup Greek Yogurt "Mayonnaise" (page 138)

1 teaspoon Dijon mustard

1. In a large pot over high heat, bring some water to a boil and add the salt.

2. Boil the potatoes for about 10 minutes until soft. Drain and cool completely.

3. In a large bowl, combine the cooled potatoes, turkey bacon, eggs, and celery.

4. In a small bowl, whisk the mayonnaise and mustard together. Toss with the potato salad until coated.

tip To mimic a fully loaded potato, eliminate the mayonnaise and mustard. Replace it with ½ cup fat-free sour cream, and add ¼ cup grated Cheddar cheese (if you tolerate it well).

PER SERVING (½ cup) Calories: 128; Total Fat: 2g; Saturated Fat: 0g; Cholesterol: 45mg; Carbohydrates: 23g; Fiber: 3g; Protein: 6g; Sodium: 230mg

Pumpkin Soup

ALKALINE **GLUTEN-FREE** **LOW-CARB** PALEO VEGAN

Serves 4
Prep: 10 minutes
Cook: 10 minutes

Earthy, savory pumpkin soup makes a delicious lunch or dinner and it's easy to put together in just 20 minutes. Be sure to use canned pumpkin purée, not pumpkin pie filling, which has added sugar and spices that would change the flavor of your soup. This is perfect for cool fall and winter days as a warming meal or snack.

2 cups Vegetable Broth (page 134)
1 (15-ounce) can pumpkin purée
1 cup unsweetened almond milk
1 teaspoon dried sage
½ teaspoon sea salt
¼ teaspoon ground nutmeg
2 tablespoons roasted pumpkin seeds

1. In a large saucepan over medium heat, stir together the broth, pumpkin purée, almond milk, sage, salt, and nutmeg.

2. Simmer for 10 minutes to allow the flavors to blend, stirring occasionally.

3. Serve garnished with the pumpkin seeds.

tip Top each bowl of soup with 1 tablespoon low-fat sour cream to add additional flavor.

PER SERVING (1 cup) Calories: 90; Total Fat: 4g; Saturated Fat: <1g; Cholesterol: 0mg; Carbohydrates: 11g; Fiber: 4g; Protein: 5g; Sodium: 667mg

Chicken Noodle Soup

Serves 4
Prep: 10 minutes
Cook: 12 minutes

Is there a food more comforting than chicken noodle soup? Traditional varieties have onion and garlic, which can definitely aggravate GERD. This version is not only acid reflux–friendly, but it is also low in carbs and gluten-free (although tradition-alists can certainly use gluten-containing noodles if they wish).

1 tablespoon extra-virgin olive oil

2 carrots, peeled and chopped

2 celery stalks, chopped

1 teaspoon dried thyme

6 cups Poultry Broth (page 132, made with chicken)

8 ounces cooked chicken breast

4 ounces pasta of choice, cooked according to package directions and drained

½ teaspoon sea salt

¼ cup fresh flat-leaf parsley, chopped

1. In a large pot over medium-high heat, heat the oil until it shimmers.

2. Add the carrots, celery, and thyme. Cook for about 6 minutes, stirring occasionally until the veggies are browned.

3. Stir in the broth. Bring to a simmer.

4. Add the chicken, pasta, and salt. Cook for 3 minutes more.

5. Stir in the parsley before serving.

tip To make this paleo and gluten-free, make zucchini noodles to replace the pasta. To make them, use a vegetable peeler to cut the zucchini lengthwise into strips, and cut the strips into smaller pieces crosswise. Sauté in 1 tablespoon olive oil for 2 minutes to heat.

tip Purchase a precooked rotisserie chicken from the grocery store. Use the breast meat (without skin) for your soup and feed the rest of the meat to your family. Alternatively, there are many excellent sources of frozen cooked chicken breast available in most grocery stores.

PER SERVING (2 cups) Calories: 503; Total Fat: 18g; Saturated Fat: 4g; Cholesterol: 176mg; Carbohydrates: 24g; Fiber: 1g; Protein: 57g; Sodium: 526mg

Cream of Mushroom Soup

ALKALINE **GLUTEN-FREE** PALEO **LOW-CARB** VEGAN

Serves 4
Prep: 10 minutes
Cook: 15 minutes

This is a favorite from my childhood, and I'm thrilled I can still enjoy it. You can use any mushrooms you like in this soup. I'm partial to shiitake mushrooms because they have such a powerful umami (savory) flavor and meaty texture.

2 tablespoons extra-virgin olive oil
8 ounces shiitake mushrooms, sliced
1 teaspoon dried thyme
½ teaspoon sea salt
6 cups Mushroom Broth (page 135)
3 tablespoons arrowroot powder
1 cup unsweetened almond milk

1. In a large pot over medium-high heat, heat the oil until it shimmers.

2. Add the mushrooms, thyme, and salt. Cook for 4 minutes without stirring. Continue to cook for 4 minutes more, stirring occasionally.

3. Stir in the broth, scraping the bottom of the pot with the side of a spoon to loosen any browned bits. Simmer for 5 minutes.

4. In a small bowl, whisk together the arrowroot powder and almond milk until smooth. Stir this slurry into the soup. Simmer for 1 to 2 minutes more, stirring constantly until the soup thickens.

tip A pinch of black pepper adds flavor, but proceed with caution—just add 1 or 2 grinds of pepper into the soup as it cooks.

PER SERVING (2 cups) Calories: 163; Total Fat: 10g; Saturated Fat: 2g; Cholesterol: 0mg; Carbohydrates: 11g; Fiber: 2g; Protein: 9g; Sodium: 522mg

Lentil Soup

GLUTEN-FREE

Serves 4
Prep: 10 minutes
Cook: 16 minutes

Traditional lentil soup is cooked long and slow with a ham hock, but that's just too fatty for people with acid reflux. Instead, smoky turkey bacon adds a depth of flavor to this soup that makes it both savory and delicious. You can also make this soup with peas in place of lentils if you enjoy pea soup.

1 tablespoon extra-virgin olive oil

4 turkey bacon slices, chopped

2 cups canned lentils, drained

1 carrot, peeled and chopped

1 teaspoon dried thyme

½ teaspoon dried rosemary

½ teaspoon sea salt

¼ teaspoon ground cumin

6 cups Vegetable Broth (page 134)

1. In a large saucepan over medium-high heat, heat the oil until it shimmers.

2. Add the turkey bacon. Cook for about 5 minutes, stirring occasionally until browned. With a slotted spoon, remove the bacon from the oil and set it aside.

3. To the pan, add the lentils, carrot, thyme, rosemary, salt, cumin, and broth. Bring to a simmer. Cook for 10 minutes, stirring occasionally until the carrots are soft.

4. Transfer the hot soup to a blender and process until smooth (see the tip). Serve garnished with the reserved bacon.

tip Safety is important when you purée hot liquids. When puréeing the soup in a blender, take off the blender lid's center cap, and use a folded towel or a potholder to hold the blender's lid in place while you purée. Every 10 seconds or so, allow the steam to escape by cracking the blender top so pressure doesn't build up—and don't overfill the blender. Work in batches if needed.

PER SERVING (2 cups) Calories: 454; Total Fat: 7g; Saturated Fat: 1g; Cholesterol: 10mg; Carbohydrates: 61g; Fiber: 30g; Protein: 35g; Sodium: 956mg

Turkey *and* Rice Soup

ALKALINE **GLUTEN-FREE** LOW-FODMAP

Serves 4
Prep: 10 minutes
Cook: 10 minutes

This easy recipe calls for precooked rice and precooked turkey breast to make a flavorful soup in a snap. This freezes well, so consider doubling the batch and freezing it in single-serving sizes for ready-made meals.

1 tablespoon extra-virgin olive oil
2 carrots, peeled and chopped
1 zucchini, chopped
1 tablespoon grated fresh ginger
½ teaspoon ground cumin
6 cups Poultry Broth (page 132)
8 ounces cooked skinless turkey
    breast, chopped
½ cup cooked brown rice
½ teaspoon sea salt

1. In a large pot over medium-high heat, heat the oil until it shimmers.

2. Add the carrots, zucchini, ginger, and cumin. Cook for 5 minutes, stirring occasionally.

3. Stir in the broth. Bring to a simmer.

4. Add the turkey, rice, and salt. Cook for 2 minutes more, stirring occasionally.

---

tip If you can't find cooked turkey breast, substitute 8 ounces ground turkey. Brown it in the pot before you cook the vegetables, and add the vegetables when it has browned.

PER SERVING (2 cups) Calories: 215; Total Fat: 7g; Saturated Fat: 1g; Cholesterol: 24mg; Carbohydrates: 19g; Fiber: 2g; Protein: 19g; Sodium: 942mg

Dill Tuna Salad Sandwich

ALKALINE **GLUTEN-FREE**

Serves 4
Prep: 10 minutes

The addition of dill to tuna salad adds a fresh, herbaceous flavor that elevates this sandwich beyond your typical tuna salad lunch. The hint of citrus zest also adds a brightness to this sandwich that pairs beautifully with the fish. To store leftovers or to transport it, save the tuna salad separately and add it to the bread just before you eat it.

1 (5-ounce) can water-packed tuna, drained and flaked
3 tablespoons Greek Yogurt "Mayonnaise" (page 138)
1 tablespoon chopped fresh dill
1 teaspoon grated orange zest
¼ teaspoon sea salt
4 gluten-free bread slices, toasted

1. In a medium bowl, mix the tuna, mayonnaise, dill, lemon zest, and salt.

2. Evenly divide and spread the tuna salad over 2 slices of bread. Top with the remaining 2 slices of bread. Cut in half and serve.

tip To zest citrus, your best choice is a rasp-style grater or the small holes on a box grater. Be sure you don't get any of the white part underneath the peel, known as the pith. This adds bitterness.

PER SERVING (½ sandwich) Calories: 144; Total Fat: 4g; Saturated Fat: <1g; Cholesterol: 11mg; Carbohydrates: 13g; Fiber: 2g; Protein: 14g; Sodium: 206mg

Grilled Pear *and* Swiss Sandwich

GLUTEN-FREE VEGETARIAN

Serves 2
Prep: 5 minutes
Cook: 6 minutes

If it's grilled cheese sandwich you crave, try this delicious twist with pear and low-fat Swiss cheese. This grown-up take on one of my personal childhood favorites is gooey, slightly sweet, and utterly delicious.

2 gluten-free bread slices
1 tablespoon unsalted butter, melted
2 (¼-inch-thick) pear slices
2 ounces low-fat Swiss cheese, grated

1. Brush one side of each bread slice with butter.

2. Lay the pear slices on the unbuttered side of one slice. Top with the cheese and the remaining slice of bread, buttered-side up.

3. In a nonstick sauté pan or skillet over medium-high heat, grill the sandwich for about 3 minutes per side until browned on both sides.

tip Pump up the flavor by replacing the butter with an equal amount of truffle oil, which adds an earthiness that beautifully complements the light sweetness of the pears.

PER SERVING (½ sandwich) Calories: 218; Total Fat: 12g; Saturated Fat: 6g; Cholesterol: 35mg; Carbohydrates: 15g; Fiber: 2g; Protein: 12g; Sodium: 214mg

Turkey and Cheddar Pockets

Serves 4
Prep: 10 minutes
Cook: 12 minutes

Remember Hot Pockets—fresh from the oven or microwave—from when you were a kid? They weren't the healthiest snack, but dang they tasted good! Here's a grown-up version made with Buttermilk Biscuit dough (page 49) that's also acid reflux–friendly, easy, and super delicious.

Nonstick cooking spray
½ recipe Buttermilk Biscuit dough (page 49)
All-purpose flour, for dusting
2 tablespoons Dijon mustard, divided
8 ounces sliced deli turkey breast
4 ounces fat-free Cheddar cheese, grated
1 egg, beaten

1. Preheat the oven to 425°F.

2. Spray a baking sheet with nonstick cooking spray.

3. Separate the biscuit dough into 4 equal balls. Roll each ball on a floured surface until it is about ⅜ inch thick.

4. Spread half of each piece of dough with 1½ teaspoons of mustard. Top each with 2 ounces of turkey and 1 ounce of Cheddar cheese.

5. Fold the other half of the dough over the filling, creating a turnover. With the tines of a fork, crimp and seal the edges. Place each turnover on the prepared sheet. Brush the tops with beaten egg.

6. Bake for about 12 minutes until golden brown.

tip Add 2 tablespoons finely chopped red apple to each turnover to add a sweet flavor that goes well with the salty cheese and turkey breast.

PER SERVING (1 turnover) Calories: 324; Total Fat: 14g; Saturated Fat: 8g; Cholesterol: 98mg; Carbohydrates: 27g; Fiber: <1g; Protein: 22g; Sodium: 1,144mg

Open-Faced Bacon, Lettuce, Cheese, *and* Avocado Sandwich

GLUTEN-FREE

Serves 1
Prep: 5 minutes
Cook: 4 minutes

When I was a child, my absolute favorite thing my mother *ever* made was an open-faced bacon, tomato, and cheese sandwich, with the cheese melted over the top of the bacon. There was just something about that crispy bacon and melty cheese I couldn't get enough of. As an adult, the sandwich evolved as I added creamy avocado to the mix. This is the acid reflux–friendly version.

1 slice gluten-free bread
1 teaspoon Dijon mustard
¼ avocado, mashed
2 turkey bacon slices, cooked and halved
1 ounce fat-free Cheddar cheese, grated

1. Preheat the broiler.

2. Place a wire rack on a baking sheet.

3. Spread the bread with the mustard and avocado.

4. Top with the bacon. Sprinkle the cheese over the top.

5. Broil for 3 to 4 minutes on the wire rack–lined sheet until the cheese melts.

tip Tomatoes are acidic, but some people can tolerate them. If you can, I highly recommend adding a slice of fresh, in-season tomato to this sandwich. Put it under the bacon and on top of the avocado.

PER SERVING (1 sandwich) Calories: 329; Total Fat: 21g; Saturated Fat: 8g; Cholesterol: 50mg; Carbohydrates: 17g; Fiber: 5g; Protein: 18g; Sodium: 537mg

Kale *and* White Bean Pita Sandwich

ALKALINE **GLUTEN-FREE** VEGETARIAN

Serves 2
Prep: 10 minutes

White bean spread makes a lovely back-drop for crisp vegetables in this simple, no-nonsense sandwich. One of the things I love about this sandwich is its versatility. Mix it up and use any veggies you like that don't aggravate your acid reflux.

½ cup canned white beans, drained and rinsed

1 teaspoon chopped fresh tarragon

1 teaspoon Dijon mustard

½ teaspoon grated orange zest

¼ teaspoon sea salt

1 gluten-free pita, halved

2 large kale leaves, thoroughly washed and dried

1. In a small bowl, mash together the white beans, tarragon, mustard, orange zest, and salt.

2. Spread the mixture evenly in the 2 pita halves.

3. Add 1 kale leaf to each.

tip Chop ¼ red bell pepper and add to the sandwiches for sweetness and extra flavor.

PER SERVING (½ pita sandwich) Calories: 216; Total Fat: <1g; Saturated Fat: 0g; Cholesterol: 0mg; Carbohydrates: 40g; Fiber: 8g; Protein: 14g; Sodium: 352mg

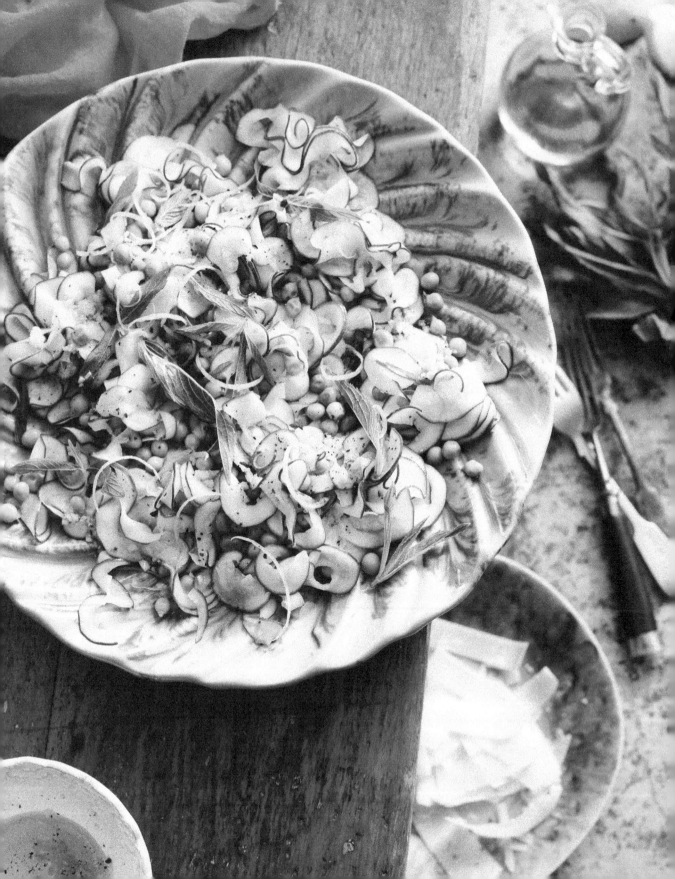

Vegetarian & Vegan

← Zucchini Noodles with Peas & Pesto, p. 85

Mini Pizzas *with* Spinach *and* White Sauce

Serves 4
Prep: 10 minutes
Cook: 12 minutes

Great news! You don't have to give up pizza if you have acid reflux. However, it may look a little different from pizzas heaped with fatty toppings and acidic tomato sauce. This lighter version is still delicious and offers the spirit of pizza without the heartburn.

4 ounces premade raw pizza dough
All-purpose flour, for dusting
½ cup Low-Fat White Sauce (page 136)
¼ cup grated fat-free Parmesan cheese
1 teaspoon dried Italian seasoning
1 cup fresh baby spinach, divided
8 mushrooms, sliced, divided
4 ounces fat-free mozzarella cheese, grated, divided
4 tablespoons chopped fresh basil

1. Preheat the oven to 400°F.

2. Divide the dough into 4 pieces. On a floured surface, roll each piece into a round that is about ³∕₈ inch thick. Place the rounds on a nonstick baking sheet.

3. In a small bowl, whisk the white sauce and Parmesan cheese together. Spread each pizza with 2 tablespoons of sauce. Sprinkle with the Italian seasoning.

4. Top each with ¼ cup of spinach, one-fourth of the mushrooms, and 1 ounce of mozzarella cheese.

5. Bake for about 12 minutes or until the dough is golden and the cheese has melted.

6. Serve garnished with the basil.

tip Add 1 tablespoon finely chopped red bell pepper to each pizza before adding the mozzarella cheese.

PER SERVING (1 pizza) Calories: 234; Total Fat: 7g; Saturated Fat: 3g; Cholesterol: 16mg; Carbohydrates: 16g; Fiber: 2g; Protein: 12g; Sodium: 801mg

Mushroom Stroganoff

ALKALINE VEGETARIAN

Serves 4
Prep: 10 minutes
Cook: 15 minutes

This warming Stroganoff is comforting and flavorful. It's long been one of my favorite meals because I love the earthiness of the mushrooms paired with the tangy sour cream and fragrant thyme. I prefer shiitake mushrooms for their savory flavor and meaty texture, but you can use any mushrooms you like.

2 tablespoons extra-virgin olive oil

12 ounces shiitake mushrooms, sliced

1 teaspoon dried thyme

½ teaspoon sea salt

3 cups Mushroom Broth (page 135)

3 tablespoons arrowroot powder

1 tablespoon Dijon mustard

½ cup fat-free sour cream

¼ cup chopped fresh parsley

6 ounces egg noodles, cooked according to package directions and drained

1. In a 12-inch nonstick sauté pan or skillet over medium-high heat, heat the oil until it shimmers.

2. Add the mushrooms, thyme, and salt. Cook for 4 minutes without stirring. Continue to cook for 4 minutes more, stirring occasionally.

3. In a small bowl, whisk together the broth, arrowroot powder, and mustard until smooth. Stir this into the mushrooms. Cook for about 2 minutes, stirring constantly until thick and warmed through.

4. Stir in the sour cream and parsley. Cook for 1 to 2 minutes, stirring constantly.

5. Serve over the hot egg noodles.

tip Make this low-carb and gluten-free by replacing the egg noodles with zucchini noodles. If you don't have a Spiralizer, use a vegetable peeler to cut the zucchini lengthwise into strips, and cut the strips into smaller pieces crosswise. Sauté in 1 tablespoon olive oil for 2 minutes to heat.

PER SERVING (1 cup sauce and ¾ cup noodles)
Calories: 250; Total Fat: 8g; Saturated Fat: 1g; Cholesterol: 15mg; Carbohydrates: 30g; Fiber: 2g; Protein: 8g; Sodium: 488mg

Fettuccine Alfredo

Serves 4
Prep: 15 minutes
Cook: 5 minutes

If it's creamy pasta you long for, you'll love this fettuccine Alfredo. Peas add a pop of green color and plenty of protein to the creamy sauce, but you can add other veggies as you wish. Try zucchini, mushrooms, or spinach to add interest and boost flavor.

3 cups (1 recipe) Low-Fat White Sauce (page 136)
1 cup cooked peas
¼ cup grated fat-free Parmesan cheese
6 ounces fettuccine noodles, cooked according to package directions and drained
2 tablespoons chopped fresh basil

1. In a medium saucepan over medium heat, simmer the white sauce, peas, and Parmesan cheese for 4 minutes, stirring constantly.

2. Toss the sauce with the hot noodles and fresh basil.

tip A little bit of red bell pepper here is a delicious and colorful addition. Finely chop ¼ red bell pepper and sauté it in 1 tablespoon olive oil for 5 minutes. Add the white sauce, peas, and Parmesan to this, and continue with the recipe as written.

PER SERVING (¼ cup sauce and 1 cup noodles)
Calories: 201; Total Fat: 2g; Saturated Fat: 1g; Cholesterol: 37mg; Carbohydrates: 33g; Fiber: 2g; Protein: 12g; Sodium: 160mg

Veggie Tacos

VEGETARIAN

Serves 4
Prep: 10 minutes
Cook: 15 minutes

Just because you have acid reflux doesn't mean Taco Tuesdays can't still be part of your week. These tasty veggie tacos are quick and easy, and they don't sacrifice flavor. Feel free to use your favorite veggies in the mix to switch it up.

4 corn tortillas
2 tablespoons extra-virgin olive oil
2 carrots, peeled and grated
1 zucchini, chopped
4 ounces mushrooms, finely chopped
1 teaspoon ground cumin
½ teaspoon ground coriander
1 teaspoon sea salt, divided
½ cup black beans, drained and heated
¼ cup chopped fresh cilantro
2 ounces fat-free Cheddar cheese, grated
½ cup fat-free sour cream
½ teaspoon grated lime zest

1. Preheat the oven to 350°F.

2. Wrap the tortillas in aluminum foil and place in the oven to warm for about 15 minutes until heated through.

3. Meanwhile, in a large nonstick sauté pan or skillet over medium-high heat, heat the oil until it shimmers.

4. Add the carrots, zucchini, mushrooms, cumin, coriander, and ½ teaspoon of salt. Cook for about 5 minutes, stirring occasionally until the vegetables begin to brown.

5. In a medium bowl, mash the black beans, cilantro, and the remaining ½ teaspoon of salt. Spread the bean mixture on the hot tortillas.

6. Top each tortilla with one-fourth of the cooked vegetables and sprinkle with Cheddar cheese.

7. In a small bowl, mix the sour cream and lime zest. Dollop on the tacos.

tip After the vegetables are cooked, add ¼ cup tomato sauce (if you tolerate it well) to the vegetables and allow it to heat through to give a little burst of tomato flavor.

PER SERVING (1 tortilla, 2 tablespoons beans, ½ cup vegetables) Calories: 236; Total Fat: 8g; Saturated Fat: 1g; Cholesterol: 6mg; Carbohydrates: 31g; Fiber: 5g; Protein: 10g; Sodium: 622mg

Quick Mushroom "Risotto"

ALKALINE **GLUTEN-FREE** VEGETARIAN

Serves 4
Prep: 10 minutes
Cook: 15 minutes

Traditional risotto takes a while to prepare, and most of the time you have to stand at the stove and stir, stir, stir. Plus, it's high in fat. This quick version comes together in less than 30 minutes using cooked brown rice, but it still has those creamy, savory flavors and textures you love.

2 tablespoons extra-virgin olive oil
4 ounces mushrooms, sliced
1 teaspoon dried thyme
½ teaspoon sea salt
1½ cups Mushroom Broth (page 135)
3 cups cooked brown rice
2 ounces fat-free cream cheese
¼ cup grated fat-free Parmesan cheese
½ cup peas, fresh or frozen

1. In a large pot over medium-high heat, heat the oil until it shimmers.

2. Add the mushrooms, thyme, and salt. Cook for 4 minutes without stirring. Continue to cook for 3 minutes more, stirring occasionally.

3. Stir in the broth and rice. Cook for about 3 minutes until the rice is warmed through.

4. Stir in the cream cheese and Parmesan cheese. Cook for about 2 minutes, stirring constantly until the cheese melts.

5. Stir in the peas. Cook for about 2 minutes more, stirring constantly until warmed through.

tip When cleaning mushrooms, don't wash them in water. They'll act like little sponges and soak it all up. Instead, wipe them carefully with a paper towel, or brush away dirt with a mushroom brush.

PER SERVING (1 cup) Calories: 449; Total Fat: 18g; Saturated Fat: 7g; Cholesterol: 26mg; Carbohydrates: 59g; Fiber: 4g; Protein: 15g; Sodium: 425mg

Zucchini Noodles *with* Peas *and* Pesto

ALKALINE **LOW-CARB** VEGETARIAN

Serves 6
Prep: 10 minutes
Cook: 5 minutes

Zucchini makes a fabulous pasta replacement for people who enjoy pasta but don't want the gluten or carbs. You can make this zucchini dish without the cheese so it's vegan and paleo (see the tip) if you wish, or leave the cheese in for a richer taste.

2 tablespoons extra-virgin olive oil
2 medium zucchini, cut lengthwise into ribbons with a vegetable peeler
1 cup peas, fresh or frozen
½ teaspoon sea salt
Zest of 1 lemon
1 cup Spinach Pesto (page 139)
Fresh basil leaves, for garnish (optional)

1. In a large sauté pan or skillet over medium-high heat, heat the oil until it shimmers.

2. Add the zucchini, peas, salt, and lemon zest.

3. Cook for 4 minutes, stirring occasionally.

4. Stir in the pesto. Garnish with the basil (if using).

tip To make this dish paleo and vegan, omit the Parmesan cheese in the Spinach Pesto recipe. Instead, add 3 tablespoons nutritional yeast.

PER SERVING (2 cups) Calories: 159;
Total Fat: 14g; Saturated Fat: 2g; Cholesterol: 2mg;
Carbohydrates: 7g; Fiber: 2g; Protein: 5g;
Sodium: 417mg

Vegetable Chow Mein

ALKALINE   VEGAN

Serves 4
Prep: 10 minutes
Cook: 12 minutes

These quick stir-fried noodles and veggies make a delicious main dish or work well as a side dish. Feel free to branch out from the veggies I suggest here, adding your own tasty flavor combinations. This recipe uses standard spaghetti noodles because they are easy to find.

2 tablespoons extra-virgin olive oil
4 ounces shiitake mushrooms, sliced
1 carrot, peeled and julienned
2 cups fresh baby spinach
6 ounces spaghetti, cooked according to package directions and drained
¼ cup Easy Ginger Stir-Fry Sauce (page 141)
1 tablespoon arrowroot powder
2 tablespoons chopped fresh cilantro

1. In a 12-inch nonstick sauté pan or skillet over medium-high heat, heat the oil until it shimmers.

2. Add the mushrooms and carrot. Cook for 5 minutes, stirring frequently.

3. Add the spinach. Cook for 2 minutes more, stirring frequently.

4. Add the cooked spaghetti and cook for 2 minutes, stirring.

5. In a small bowl, whisk the stir-fry sauce and arrowroot powder together until smooth. Add this to the pan. Cook for 1 to 2 minutes, stirring constantly until thick.

6. Remove from the heat and stir in the cilantro.

tip   To make this paleo, low carb, and gluten-free, replace the spaghetti with zucchini noodles. If you don't have a Spiralizer, use a vegetable peeler to cut the zucchini lengthwise into strips, and cut the strips into smaller pieces crosswise. Sauté in 1 tablespoon olive oil for 2 minutes to heat.

tip   If you can't find arrowroot powder, cornstarch works as well.

PER SERVING (1½ cups) Calories: 217; Total Fat: 8g; Saturated Fat: 1g; Cholesterol: 31mg; Carbohydrates: 31g; Fiber: 2g; Protein: 7g; Sodium: 553mg

Edamame Stir-Fry

ALKALINE VEGAN

Serves 4
Prep: 10 minutes
Cook: 10 minutes

Edamame is a great vegan source of protein, and it's a rock star as the main ingredient in this delicious stir-fry. Serve it over brown rice to soak up the flavorful sauce. This freezes well, so it's a great way to make meals ahead of time. Store it in single-serving sizes in freezer containers for meals on the go.

2 tablespoons extra-virgin olive oil
2 cups edamame, fresh or frozen and thawed
2 cups chopped kale
1 cup peas, fresh or frozen and thawed
2 large carrots, peeled and julienned
4 ounces sliced mushrooms
1 tablespoon grated fresh ginger
¼ cup Easy Ginger Stir-Fry Sauce (page 141)
1 tablespoon arrowroot powder
Zest of 1 lime
2 cups cooked brown rice

1. In a 12-inch nonstick sauté pan or skillet over medium-high heat, heat the oil until it shimmers.

2. Add the edamame, kale, peas, carrots, mushrooms, and ginger. Cook for 5 minutes, stirring frequently.

3. In a small bowl, whisk together the stir-fry sauce, arrowroot powder, and lime zest. Add this to the vegetables and cook for 1 to 2 minutes, stirring constantly until it thickens.

4. Serve over the rice.

tip If you can't find fresh or frozen edamame, replace it with an equal amount of peas or lentils.

PER SERVING (2 cups vegetables with ½ cup rice) Calories: 369; Total Fat: 8g; Saturated Fat: 1g; Cholesterol: 0mg; Carbohydrates: 63g; Fiber: 8g; Protein: 13g; Sodium: 755mg

Lentils and Couscous

Serves 4
Prep: 10 minutes
Cook: 11 minutes

Lentils are a tasty source of protein for vegan diets. Combining them with couscous provides a grain and a legume, which makes a complete protein. You'll enjoy this warming, flavorful dish. It freezes well for meals on the go—whip up a double batch and keep some nutritious meals stocked for those busy nights.

2 tablespoons extra-virgin olive oil
2 carrots, peeled and chopped
3 cups canned lentils, drained
2 teaspoons dried tarragon
Zest of 1 orange
½ teaspoon sea salt
2 cups whole-wheat couscous, cooked according to package directions and drained

1. In a large saucepan over medium-high heat, heat the oil until it shimmers.

2. Add the carrots. Cook for about 5 minutes, stirring occasionally until soft.

3. Add the lentils, tarragon, orange zest, and salt. Cook for 5 minutes, stirring occasionally.

4. Stir in the couscous and serve.

tip Want to add a big pop of flavor and color? Replace the carrots with 2 beets, peeled and diced.

PER SERVING (2 cups) Calories: 500;
Total Fat: 9g; Saturated Fat: 1g; Cholesterol: 0mg;
Carbohydrates: 82g; Fiber: 27g; Protein: 26g;
Sodium: 272mg

Easy Asparagus Quiche Bites

ALKALINE **LOW-CARB** VEGETARIAN

Serves 6
Prep: 5 minutes
Cook: 25 minutes

Baking a quiche takes time, but if you divide the batter up in a muffin tin, it cooks a lot more quickly. These single-serving quiches are loaded with flavor, cook quickly, and freeze well. Make a double batch and freeze in a zip-top bag. Heat in the microwave to enjoy a meal on the go.

Nonstick cooking spray
2 tablespoons extra-virgin olive oil
6 asparagus spears, trimmed and chopped
8 eggs, beaten
¼ cup unsweetened almond milk
1 teaspoon dried thyme
½ teaspoon sea salt
2 ounces fat-free cheese of choice, grated

1. Preheat the oven to 350°F.

2. Spray a 6-muffin tin with nonstick cooking spray.

3. In a large saucepan over medium-high heat, heat the oil until it shimmers.

4. Add the asparagus. Cook for about 5 minutes, stirring occasionally until soft. Let cool.

5. Meanwhile, in a medium bowl, whisk the eggs, almond milk, thyme, and salt together until well combined.

6. Fold in the asparagus and cheese. Evenly divide among the muffin tins.

7. Bake for about 20 minutes until set.

tip   To trim asparagus, hold each spear lightly at each end and bend it until it snaps. Discard the thick, woody end and chop the tender pieces.

PER SERVING (1 "muffin") Calories: 168; Total Fat: 13g; Saturated Fat: 5g; Cholesterol: 221mg; Carbohydrates: 3g; Fiber: <1g; Protein: 10g; Sodium: 393mg

Cheesy Broccoli *and* Cauliflower Bake

Serves 4
Prep: 10 minutes
Cook: 5 minutes

Here's a lower-carb version of mac 'n' cheese—minus the mac but with tasty veggies instead. This is a delicious main dish, or it's fantastic as a side dish or snack. It's also a showstopper at parties, so bring some along to share as your secret weapon for fighting acid reflux while you socialize.

3 cups (1 recipe) Low-Fat White Sauce (page 136)
2 ounces fat-free sharp Cheddar cheese, grated
2 cups broccoli florets, steamed
2 cups cauliflower florets, steamed
¼ cup bread crumbs
1 tablespoon unsalted butter, melted

1. Preheat the broiler to high.

2. In a medium saucepan over medium-low heat, cook the white sauce and Cheddar cheese for 2 to 3 minutes, whisking constantly until the cheese melts.

3. Stir in the broccoli and cauliflower. Evenly divide among four (6-ounce) ramekins.

4. In a small bowl, combine the bread crumbs and butter. Sprinkle evenly over the ramekins.

5. Broil for 1 to 2 minutes until the bread crumbs are golden.

tip To steam broccoli and cauliflower, place in a steamer basket in a saucepan filled with about 1 inch of water. Cover and steam until tender, 5 to 10 minutes.

PER SERVING (1 ramekin) Calories: 134;
Total Fat: 5g; Saturated Fat: 3g; Cholesterol: 16mg;
Carbohydrates: 16g; Fiber: 3g; Protein: 9g;
Sodium: 479mg

Zucchini Lasagna *with* White Sauce

ALKALINE **GLUTEN-FREE** **LOW-CARB** VEGETARIAN

Serves 6
Prep: 10 minutes
Cook: 20 minutes

Craving lasagna? I get it. With my celiac disease, I've had to come up with all sorts of clever ways to make lasagna I can eat, and this is one of them. Making these simple lasagnas in muffin cups allows them to cook quickly. You can pop them out of the tins and freeze them in zip-top bags for quick meals later.

Nonstick cooking spray

1½ cups fat-free ricotta cheese

¼ cup Spinach Pesto (page 139)

1½ cups Low-Fat White Sauce
(page 136), divided

2 medium zucchini, thinly sliced, divided

6 tablespoons grated fat-free mozzarella
cheese, divided

1. Preheat the oven to 350°F.

2. Spray a 6-muffin tin with nonstick cooking spray.

3. In a small bowl, mix the ricotta cheese and pesto.

4. Spread 1 tablespoon of white sauce in the bottom of each muffin cup. Evenly divide half the zucchini slices among the cups.

5. Top with equal amounts of the ricotta and pesto mixture. Top again with the remaining zucchini slices.

6. Cover each with equal amounts of the remaining white sauce and 1 tablespoon of mozzarella cheese.

7. Bake for 20 minutes until the cheese is bubbly.

tip Stir ¼ cup tomato sauce (if you tolerate it well) into the white sauce to give it a rich tomato flavor.

PER SERVING (1 "muffin") Calories: 172;
Total Fat: 10g; Saturated Fat: 5g; Cholesterol: 27mg;
Carbohydrates: 8g; Fiber: <1g; Protein: 12g;
Sodium: 438mg

Tofu *and* Vegetable Scramble

ALKALINE   **GLUTEN-FREE**   **LOW-CARB**   VEGAN

Serves 4
Prep: 10 minutes
Cook: 11 minutes

This is a good vegan breakfast if you're not an egg fan, and it makes a tasty main dish for lunch or dinner. My favorite type of tofu is silken tofu because I like the texture, but you may use any that you like. The trick to flavorful tofu is to remove the water (see the tip) before mixing it with other flavors.

2 tablespoons extra-virgin olive oil
1 (12-ounce) package silken tofu, cubed
8 ounces mushrooms, sliced
1 zucchini, sliced
1 teaspoon dried rosemary
2 tablespoons gluten-free soy sauce
1 tablespoon Dijon mustard
1 tablespoon grated orange zest

1. In a 12-inch nonstick sauté pan or skillet over medium-high heat, heat the oil until it shimmers.

2. Add the tofu, mushrooms, zucchini, and rosemary. Cook for about 7 minutes, stirring occasionally until the veggies begin to brown.

3. In a small bowl, whisk together the soy sauce, mustard, and orange zest. Add to the stir-fry. Cook for 3 minutes more, stirring occasionally.

tip To remove water from tofu, place the tofu between paper towels or clean kitchen towels. Let sit for 10 minutes for excess water to drain.

PER SERVING (1½ cups) Calories: 147; Total Fat: 11g; Saturated Fat: 2g; Cholesterol: 0mg; Carbohydrates: 6g; Fiber: 2g; Protein: 10g; Sodium: 514mg

Quick Tofu, Carrot, *and* Mushroom Stir-Fry

ALKALINE **GLUTEN-FREE** VEGAN

Serves 4
Prep: 10 minutes
Cook: 10 minutes

An easy and quick meal in 10 minutes—what could be better? Save time by reheating precooked brown rice you've purchased or made yourself and you will have the perfect, protein-packed vegan meal for a busy weeknight.

2 tablespoons extra-virgin olive oil

1 (12-ounce) package silken tofu, cubed

8 ounces mushrooms, sliced

3 carrots, peeled and sliced

1 cup (1 recipe) Easy Ginger Stir-Fry Sauce (page 141)

2 tablespoons arrowroot powder

¼ cup chopped fresh cilantro

2 cups cooked brown rice, hot

1. In a 12-inch nonstick sauté pan or skillet over medium-high heat, heat the oil until it shimmers.

2. Add the tofu, mushrooms, and carrots. Cook for about 7 minutes, stirring occasionally until the veggies begin to brown.

3. In a small bowl, whisk together the stir-fry sauce and arrowroot powder. Add this to the pan. Cook for about 2 minutes more, stirring occasionally until thickened.

4. Remove from the heat and stir in the cilantro. Serve with the rice.

tip Not a cilantro fan? Many people aren't because they have a genetic predisposition that causes it to taste soapy. If this describes you, replace it with chopped fresh basil, or eliminate it altogether.

PER SERVING (1½ cups tofu and veggies with ½ cup rice) Calories: 334; Total Fat: 12g; Saturated Fat: 2g; Cholesterol: 0mg; Carbohydrates: 46g; Fiber: 4g; Protein: 14g; Sodium: 949mg

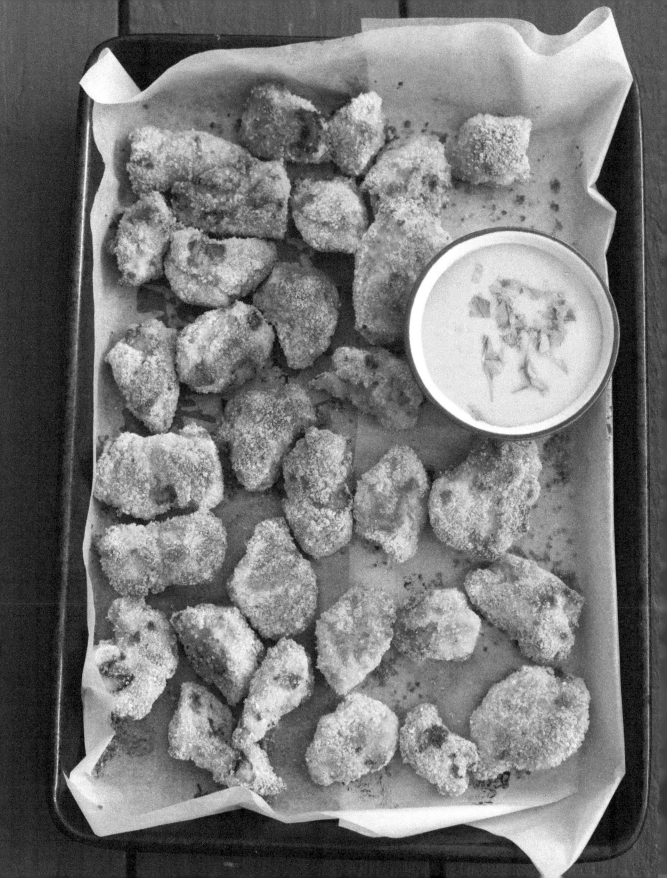

Poultry & Pork

"Fried" Chicken with Country Gravy

Serves 4
Prep: 10 minutes
Cook: 15 minutes

While fried chicken usually takes a long time to make, pounding chicken breast tenders into thin cutlets and baking them goes quickly—and without the deep-fried coating, triggering acid reflux is far less likely. Serve with a side of Sweet Potato Oven "Fries" (page 54).

FOR THE CHICKEN

1 cup all-purpose flour
1 tablespoon sea salt
1 teaspoon dried thyme
2 eggs, beaten
2 tablespoons unsweetened almond milk
4 (3-ounce) boneless skinless chicken breast tenders, pounded ⅜ inch thick
2 tablespoons unsalted butter

TO MAKE THE CHICKEN

1. Preheat the oven to 200°F.

2. Line a baking sheet with a wire rack.

3. In a shallow dish, whisk the flour, salt, and thyme together.

4. In another shallow dish, whisk together the eggs and almond milk.

5. Dip the chicken pieces into the flour and tap off any excess. Dip them into the egg mixture and back into the flour to coat, tapping off any excess flour.

6. In a 12-inch nonstick sauté pan or skillet over medium-high heat, melt the butter until it bubbles.

7. Add the coated chicken and cook for 3 to 4 minutes per side or until done. Transfer the chicken to the rack on the baking sheet and place it into the oven to keep warm.

FOR THE GRAVY

1 tablespoon unsalted butter

3 tablespoons all-purpose flour

1 cup Mushroom Broth (page 135)

1 cup unsweetened almond milk

½ teaspoon sea salt

Pinch freshly ground black pepper

TO MAKE THE GRAVY

1. In the pan you used to cook the chicken, over medium-high heat, melt the butter until it bubbles.

2. Whisk in the flour and cook for 2 minutes, whisking constantly.

3. Stir in the broth, almond milk, salt, and pepper. Cook for about 2 minutes more, stirring constantly until the gravy thickens.

tip To pound the chicken flat, place each piece between two pieces of parchment paper or plastic wrap and use a mallet to pound to ⅜ inch thick.

PER SERVING (1 cutlet with ¼ cup gravy)
Calories: 439; Total Fat: 18g; Saturated Fat: 8g; Cholesterol: 180mg; Carbohydrates: 36g; Fiber: 1g; Protein: 31g; Sodium: 1,516mg

Chicken Nuggets *with* Honey Mustard Dipping Sauce

GLUTEN-FREE

Serves 4
Prep: 10 minutes
Cook: 20 minutes

These oven-baked chicken nuggets are coated in tasty, seasoned bread crumbs that are so delicious, you won't even miss the deep-frying. Serve them with Baked Green Bean "Fries" (page 52), Baked Potato Chips (page 53), or Creamy Coleslaw (page 65) for a reflux-friendly comfort food meal.

Nonstick cooking spray

1 cup gluten-free bread crumbs

1 tablespoon sea salt

1 teaspoon dried thyme

1 teaspoon dried rosemary

2 eggs, beaten

1 cup unsweetened almond milk

4 (3-ounce) boneless skinless chicken breast tenders, cut into ¾-inch pieces

½ cup Honey Mustard Dipping Sauce (page 98)

1. Preheat the oven to 425°F.

2. Spray a baking sheet with nonstick cooking spray.

3. In a shallow dish, mix the bread crumbs, salt, thyme, and rosemary.

4. In another shallow dish, whisk together the eggs and almond milk.

5. Dip the chicken pieces into the egg mixture and into the seasoned bread crumbs to coat, tapping off any excess coating. Place the nuggets on the prepared sheet.

6. Bake for about 20 minutes until the bread crumbs are golden and the chicken is cooked through.

7. Serve with the dipping sauce.

tip Add ⅛ teaspoon freshly ground black pepper (if you tolerate it well) to the bread crumbs to boost flavor.

PER SERVING (3 ounces chicken with 2 tablespoons sauce) Calories: 340; Total Fat: 10g; Saturated Fat: 3g; Cholesterol: 158mg; Carbohydrates: 28g; Fiber: 1g; Protein: 34g; Sodium: 893mg

Turkey Sliders

GLUTEN-FREE LOW-CARB

Serves 8
Prep: 14 minutes
Cook: 8 to 16 minutes

Sometimes it just has be a burger—but not that greasy, fatty, acid reflux–inviting kind. When the craving hits, give these tasty sliders a try. They have a slightly sweet and savory sauce that's delicious, and the small size is the perfect portion to prevent you from experiencing an acid reflux flare-up, especially when you serve it with a side of Potato Salad (page 67).

1 pound ground turkey breast
2 teaspoons dried thyme
1 teaspoon packed brown sugar
½ teaspoon fish sauce
½ teaspoon sea salt
Nonstick cooking spray
8 gluten-free slider buns
½ cup Umami Burger Sauce (page 140)

1. In a large bowl, mix the turkey, thyme, brown sugar, fish sauce, and salt. Form into 8 patties.

2. Spray a 12-inch skillet with nonstick cooking spray and place over medium-high heat.

3. Add the patties (working in batches if needed) and cook for about 4 minutes per side, until the meat is cooked through.

4. Place each patty on a bun. Top each with 1 tablespoon of burger sauce.

tip There are many kinds of ground turkey with varying degrees of fat—some include dark meat and some have the skin ground up in them. Choose a ground turkey that is breast meat only, no skin. You'll be able to tell because the color is very light, the same color as raw turkey breast. Darker ground turkey is likely to contain skin and dark meat.

PER SERVING (1 slider and bun with 1 tablespoon sauce) Calories: 196; Total Fat: 6g; Saturated Fat: 2g; Cholesterol: 42mg; Carbohydrates: 16g; Fiber: 7g; Protein: 20g; Sodium: 410mg

Kale *and* Herb–Stuffed Turkey Cutlets

ALKALINE   **GLUTEN-FREE**   **LOW-CARB**   PALEO

Serves 4
Prep: 15 minutes
Cook: 12 minutes

Love stuffed turkey? It's a seasonal favorite, but Thanksgiving can be an acid reflux attack just waiting to happen with all the rich, fatty foods and big portions. While you can make this lightened version of stuffed turkey any time of year, it makes a great stand-in for that blowout Thanksgiving meal and will leave you free of acid reflux.

2 tablespoons extra-virgin olive oil
½ bunch kale, trimmed and cut into pieces
1 teaspoon dried thyme
1 teaspoon sea salt, divided
4 (3-ounce) pieces turkey breast, pounded ⅜ inch thick
1 cup Mushroom Gravy (page 143), warmed

1. In a 12-inch nonstick sauté pan or skillet over medium-high heat, heat the oil until it shimmers.

2. Add the kale, thyme, and ½ teaspoon of salt. Cook for about 5 minutes, stirring occasionally until the kale is soft. Remove the kale from the pan and set it aside. Return the pan to the heat.

3. Season the turkey with the remaining ½ teaspoon of salt. Add it to the pan and cook for about 3 minutes per side until it is cooked through.

4. Top each piece of turkey with one-fourth of the kale. Roll the turkey around the kale. Top each with ¼ cup of gravy.

tip When you sauté the kale, add ½ red bell pepper, finely chopped, to add flavor, color, and texture.

PER SERVING (3 ounces turkey, ¼ cup kale, ¼ cup gravy) Calories: 203; Total Fat: 9g; Saturated Fat: 2g; Cholesterol: 40mg; Carbohydrates: 12g; Fiber: 2g; Protein: 18g; Sodium: 1,491mg

Turkey *and* Sweet Potatoes

ALKALINE **GLUTEN-FREE** PALEO

Serves 4
Prep: 7 minutes
Cook: 23 minutes

Here's another tasty Thanksgiving stand-in. Sweet potatoes are quickly sautéed and glazed with honey, which is a nice change from the candied sweet potatoes at Thanksgiving. It's a truly delicious and satisfying meal.

4 (3-ounce) pieces turkey breast, pounded ⅜ inch thick

1 teaspoon sea salt, divided

2 tablespoons extra-virgin olive oil, divided

1 large sweet potato, peeled and cut into ½-inch cubes

1 teaspoon dried thyme

2 tablespoons honey

1 teaspoon grated orange zest

1. Season the turkey with $\frac{1}{2}$ teaspoon of salt.

2. In a 12-inch nonstick sauté pan or skillet over medium-high heat, heat 1 tablespoon of oil until it shimmers.

3. Add the turkey and cook for about 3 minutes per side until browned and cooked through. Transfer to a plate, tent loosely with aluminum foil to keep it warm, and set it aside. Return the pan to the heat.

4. Heat the remaining 1 tablespoon of oil in the pan. Add the sweet potato, thyme, and the remaining $\frac{1}{2}$ teaspoon of salt. Cook for 10 to 15 minutes, stirring occasionally until the potatoes have browned.

5. Stir in the honey and orange zest. Cook for 1 minute more, stirring constantly.

tip   To make this low-FODMAP, omit the honey and use less than ½ cup of sweet potato.

PER SERVING (3 ounces turkey and ¼ cup sweet potatoes) Calories: 222; Total Fat: 9g; Saturated Fat: 1g; Cholesterol: 37mg; Carbohydrates: 22g; Fiber: 2g; Protein: 16g; Sodium: 544mg

Chicken à la King

Serves 4
Prep: 15 minutes
Cook: 15 minutes

This creamy chicken dish is a favorite for many with its rich mushroom sauce and flavorful chicken topping buttered egg noodles. The original version, however, is high in acid reflux–causing ingredients, including lots of fat and green peppers. This version tastes just as good and retains the spirit of the original, without the heartburn.

2 tablespoons extra-virgin olive oil, divided

8 ounces mushrooms, sliced

8 ounces boneless skinless chicken breast, cut into ½-inch dice

½ teaspoon sea salt

1 cup peas, fresh or frozen and thawed

2 cups Mushroom Gravy (page 143)

¼ cup chopped fresh parsley

8 ounces egg noodles, cooked according to package directions and drained

1. In a 12-inch nonstick sauté pan or skillet over medium-high heat, heat 1 tablespoon of oil until it shimmers.

2. Add the mushrooms. Cook for 5 minutes, stirring once or twice. Transfer to a plate and set it aside. Return the pan to the heat.

3. Heat the remaining 1 tablespoon of oil in the pan. Add the chicken and cook for about 5 minutes, stirring occasionally until cooked through.

4. Stir the mushrooms back into the pan. Add the salt, peas, and gravy. Cook for about 2 minutes, stirring frequently until the peas are heated through.

5. Stir in the parsley.

6. Serve over the egg noodles.

tip Add color and extra flavor by dicing ½ red bell pepper and cooking it with the mushrooms.

PER SERVING (1 cup sauce and 1 cup egg noodles) Calories: 318; Total Fat: 11g; Saturated Fat: 3g; Cholesterol: 66mg; Carbohydrates: 27g; Fiber: 3g; Protein: 27g; Sodium: 676mg

Turkey Noodle Casserole

Serves 4
Prep: 14 minutes
Cook: 16 minutes

If you like the idea of tuna noodle casserole but don't like tuna, try this turkey take on it. It's easy to make, and the creamy, flavorful sauce tastes rich but doesn't have the fat to cause acid reflux.

8 ounces ground turkey breast

2 tablespoons extra-virgin olive oil

8 ounces mushrooms, sliced

2 cups Mushroom Gravy (page 143)

1 cup peas, fresh or frozen and thawed

1 tablespoon soy sauce

3 cups rotini pasta, cooked according to
    package directions and drained

½ cup bread crumbs

1 tablespoon unsalted butter, melted

1. Preheat the broiler to medium-high.

2. In a 12-inch nonstick sauté pan or skillet over medium-high heat, brown the turkey for about 5 minutes, crumbling it with a spoon until done. Remove the turkey from the pan and set it aside. Return the pan to the heat.

3. Heat the oil in the pan until it shimmers. Add the mushrooms. Cook for 5 minutes, stirring once or twice.

4. Stir in the gravy, peas, soy sauce, and reserved turkey. Cook for about 3 minutes, stirring constantly until the peas are warm. Stir in the hot pasta.

5. Evenly divide the casserole among four (6-ounce) ramekins.

6. In a small bowl, mix the bread crumbs and butter. Sprinkle over the ramekins.

7. Broil for about 2 minutes until the bread crumbs have browned.

tip Stir in ¼ cup grated fat-free sharp Cheddar cheese (if you tolerate it well) when you add the pasta.

PER SERVING (1 ramekin) Calories: 437;
Total Fat: 20g; Saturated Fat: 6g; Cholesterol: 96mg;
Carbohydrates: 39g; Fiber: 3.3g; Protein: 29g;
Sodium: 690mg

Easy Turkey Meatloaf "Muffins"

ALKALINE **LOW-CARB** PALEO

Serves 6
Prep: 5 minutes
Cook: 25 minutes

Cooking meatloaf as muffins instead of in a big loaf pan has two advantages: portion control and quicker cooking time. It will take about 30 minutes for these to come together, but most of that is inactive time when you can enjoy the lovely scents filling your home.

18 ounces ground turkey breast
3 carrots, peeled and grated
1 egg, beaten
1 tablespoon soy sauce
1 tablespoon Dijon mustard
1 teaspoon fish sauce
1 teaspoon dried thyme
1 teaspoon dried rosemary

1. Preheat the oven to 350°F.

2. In a large bowl, mix the turkey, carrots, egg, soy sauce, mustard, fish sauce, thyme, and rosemary well. Evenly divide the meatloaf mixture among the cups of a nonstick 6-muffin tin.

3. Bake for about 25 minutes until cooked through.

tip Spread 1 teaspoon tomato sauce over each meatloaf before baking.

PER SERVING (1 "muffin") Calories: 188; Total Fat: 7g; Saturated Fat: 2g; Cholesterol: 90mg; Carbohydrates: 4g; Fiber: 1g; Protein: 26g; Sodium: 342mg

Mini Pizzas with Canadian Bacon and White Sauce

Serves 4
Prep: 15 minutes
Cook: 12 minutes

Like pizza? You're not alone. Americans eat about 350 slices of pizza per minute every single day, and over five billion pizzas are sold annually worldwide, according to Pizza.com. Don't get left out! Make your own GERD-friendly pizza with this simple, quick, and delicious recipe.

Nonstick cooking spray
4 ounces premade raw pizza dough
All-purpose flour, for dusting
½ cup Low-Fat White Sauce (page 136)
¼ cup grated fat-free Parmesan cheese
8 ounces Canadian bacon, cut into pieces
4 ounces fat-free mozzarella cheese, grated
4 fresh basil leaves, finely chopped

1. Preheat the oven to 400°F.

2. Spray a baking sheet with nonstick cooking spray.

3. Divide the dough into 4 pieces. On a floured surface, roll out each piece until it is ½ inch thick. Place the rounds on the prepared sheet.

4. In a small bowl, stir together the white sauce and Parmesan cheese. Spread each dough round with 2 tablespoons of the white sauce and cheese mixture.

5. Top each with equal amounts of Canadian bacon and mozzarella cheese.

6. Bake for about 12 minutes or until the dough is crisp and the cheese is melted and bubbly.

7. Sprinkle with the basil before serving.

tip   Add 1 tablespoon chopped red bell pepper to each pizza on top of the Canadian bacon before adding the mozzarella cheese.

PER SERVING (1 pizza) Calories: 176; Total Fat: 5g; Saturated Fat: 2g; Cholesterol: 38mg; Carbohydrates: 11g; Fiber: 0g; Protein: 20g; Sodium: 1,729mg

Soba Noodle *and* Ground Turkey Stir-Fry

ALKALINE

Serves 4
Prep: 10 minutes
Cook: 15 minutes

Soba noodles are a Japanese noodle made from buckwheat flour. They are great in stir-fries and make a nice alternative to rice. So, if you're craving Asian take-out food, try this tasty, quick stir-fry instead. It will satisfy your craving without aggravating your GERD.

2 tablespoons extra-virgin olive oil
8 ounces ground turkey breast
8 ounces shiitake mushrooms, sliced
3 carrots, peeled and sliced
2 cups fresh baby spinach
¼ cup Easy Ginger Stir-Fry Sauce (page 141)
½ teaspoon toasted sesame oil
4 ounces soba noodles, cooked according to package directions and drained
2 tablespoons chopped fresh cilantro

1. In a 12-inch nonstick sauté pan or skillet over medium-high heat, heat the olive oil until it shimmers.

2. Add the turkey. Cook for about 5 minutes, stirring occasionally and crumbling it with a spoon until browned. With a slotted spoon, remove the turkey from the oil and set it aside. Return the pan to the heat.

3. In the same pan, cook the mushrooms and carrots for about 5 minutes, stirring occasionally until soft.

4. Add the spinach and cook for 2 minutes more.

5. Return the turkey to the pan, along with the stir-fry sauce, sesame oil, and noodles. Simmer for 2 minutes to warm through.

6. Stir in the cilantro.

tip Sprinkle sesame seeds (if you tolerate them well) over each portion—about ½ teaspoon each.

PER SERVING (2 cups) Calories: 262; Total Fat: 9g; Saturated Fat: 1g; Cholesterol: 24mg; Carbohydrates: 32g; Fiber: 2g; Protein: 17g; Sodium: 1,116mg

Chicken, Mushroom, *and* Rice Casserole

ALKALINE **GLUTEN-FREE**

Serves 4
Prep: 7 minutes
Cook: 23 minutes

When I was a child, my mom made a casserole she called "company chicken." It was, essentially, a baked combination of cream of mushroom soup, chicken, pearl onions, mushrooms, cheese, and rice. I loved that stuff, and everyone else seemed to love it as well. With so many GERD triggers in a single dish, however, it wasn't something I could bring along as an adult, so I made my own version.

2 tablespoons extra-virgin olive oil
6 ounces boneless skinless chicken breast, chopped
8 ounces mushrooms, sliced
2 cups Mushroom Gravy (page 143)
½ teaspoon sea salt
½ cup grated fat-free Cheddar cheese
2 cups cooked white rice

1. Preheat the oven to 350°F.

2. In a 12-inch nonstick sauté pan or skillet over medium-high heat, heat the oil until it shimmers.

3. Add the chicken. Cook for about 5 minutes, stirring occasionally until cooked. With a slotted spoon, remove the chicken from the oil and set it aside. Return the pan to the heat.

4. Add the mushrooms to the pan and cook for 5 minutes, stirring once or twice.

5. Return the chicken to the pan along with the gravy and salt. Simmer for 2 minutes to warm. Remove from the heat.

6. Fold in the Cheddar cheese and rice. Spoon the mixture evenly into four (6- to 8-ounce) ramekins.

7. Bake for 10 minutes or until the cheese melts.

tip Use any fat-free cheese you prefer. I enjoy sharp Cheddar, but Swiss works well, too.

PER SERVING (1 ramekin) Calories: 576; Total Fat: 20g; Saturated Fat: 5g; Cholesterol: 126mg; Carbohydrates: 47g; Fiber: 1g; Protein: 50g; Sodium: 854mg

White Bean, Chicken, *and* Rosemary Casserole

ALKALINE **GLUTEN-FREE**

Serves 4
Prep: 10 minutes
Cook: 20 minutes

French *cassoulet* is a decadent combination of white beans with duck confit. It's an explosion of flavor—and fat and acid. This lightened version offers similar flavor profiles but with far fewer consequences to those of us with acid reflux. It's also quick and easy.

8 ounces cooked boneless skinless
    chicken breast
2 cups canned white beans, drained
2 cups Mushroom Gravy (page 143)
2 teaspoons dried rosemary
½ teaspoon sea salt

1. Preheat the oven to 350°F.

2. In a large bowl, mix the chicken, beans, gravy, rosemary, and salt. Spoon the mixture evenly into four (6- to 8-ounce) ramekins.

3. Bake for 20 minutes.

tip Sprinkle 1 tablespoon grated Parmesan cheese (if you tolerate it well) on top of each ramekin before baking.

PER SERVING (1 ramekin) Calories: 565; Total Fat: 16g; Saturated Fat: 5g; Cholesterol: 160mg; Carbohydrates: 37g; Fiber: 8g; Protein: 66g; Sodium: 671mg

Pan-Seared Pork Tenderloin
with Mustard-Rosemary Pan Sauce

ALKALINE **GLUTEN-FREE** **LOW-CARB** LOW-FODMAP PALEO

Serves 4
Prep: 10 minutes
Cook: 15 minutes

Pork and mustard have a natural affinity, and this recipe takes advantage of that. Tenderloin is a wonderful, lean substitute for higher-fat pork chops, and the quick pan-sear keeps fat low and flavor high. Enjoy it with Roasted Parmesan Potatoes (page 55) for a hearty and satisfying meal.

12 ounces pork tenderloin, cut into
    ½-inch-thick pieces
1 teaspoon sea salt, divided
2 tablespoons unsalted butter, divided
1 cup Poultry Broth (page 132)
1 tablespoon Dijon mustard
2 tablespoons chopped fresh rosemary

1. Season the pork with ½ teaspoon of salt.

2. In a 12-inch nonstick sauté pan or skillet over medium-high heat, melt 1 tablespoon of butter until it bubbles.

3. Add the pork. Cook for about 4 minutes per side until done. Transfer to a plate and tent loosely with aluminum foil. Return the pan to the heat.

4. To the pan, add the broth, mustard, rosemary, and remaining ½ teaspoon of salt. Cook for about 5 minutes, whisking occasionally until the liquid has reduced by half. Whisk in the remaining 1 tablespoon of butter until it is just melted and incorporated.

5. Serve the tenderloin pieces with the sauce spooned over the top.

tip When searing pork tenderloin, leave it in contact with the pan for as long as possible without moving it. This allows the sugars on the surface of the meat to caramelize, adding a deep, rich flavor.

PER SERVING (3 ounces pork with ¼ cup sauce)
Calories: 190; Total Fat: 10g; Saturated Fat: 5g; Cholesterol: 77mg; Carbohydrates: 2g; Fiber: <1g; Protein: 24g; Sodium: 620mg

Pasta Carbonara

Serves 4
Prep: 15 minutes
Cook: 8 minutes

Pasta carbonara is just a fancy way of saying bacon-and-egg pasta. This flavorful dish is so satisfying, quick, and delicious. It's something I can whip together in my kitchen in about 20 minutes, so it's a perfect speedy meal for a busy weeknight.

2 tablespoons extra-virgin olive oil
8 turkey bacon slices, chopped
1 cup peas, fresh or frozen and thawed
½ cup Mushroom Broth (page 135)
½ teaspoon sea salt
8 ounces spaghetti, cooked according to package directions and drained
4 eggs, beaten
1 tablespoon heavy (whipping) cream
2 tablespoons grated fat-free Parmesan cheese

1. In a 12-inch nonstick sauté pan or skillet over medium-high heat, heat the oil until it shimmers.

2. Add the turkey bacon. Cook for about 4 minutes, stirring occasionally until browned.

3. Stir in the peas, broth, and salt. Bring to a simmer.

4. Add the spaghetti.

5. In a small bowl, whisk the eggs and heavy cream together. Stir the eggs into the hot pan, cooking and stirring for 30 seconds.

6. Sprinkle in the Parmesan cheese and serve.

tip You can replace the turkey bacon with 2 ounces pancetta.

PER SERVING (1 cup noodles with ½ cup sauce)
Calories: 385; Total Fat: 16g; Saturated Fat: 4g; Cholesterol: 232mg; Carbohydrates: 37g; Fiber: 2g; Protein: 22g; Sodium: 620mg

Chicken *and* Fennel Sauté

ALKALINE **GLUTEN-FREE** **LOW-CARB** PALEO

Serves 4
Prep: 5 minutes
Cook: 8 minutes

Fennel has a lovely anise flavor, and many people find that its alkalinity is beneficial to GERD. This dish is quick and tasty, and you can serve it alone or with your favorite side dish—or even a simple salad. It's an easy dinner for busy weeknights.

2 tablespoons extra-virgin olive oil

1 fennel bulb, thinly sliced

12 ounces boneless skinless chicken breast, chopped into ½-inch pieces

½ teaspoon sea salt

½ cup Poultry Broth (page 132)

1 teaspoon Dijon mustard

1 teaspoon dried thyme

1 teaspoon grated orange zest

1. In a 12-inch nonstick sauté pan or skillet over medium-high heat, heat the oil until it shimmers.

2. Add the fennel, chicken, and salt. Cook for about 5 minutes, stirring occasionally until the chicken is cooked through.

3. In a small bowl, whisk together the broth, mustard, thyme, and orange zest. Stir this into the chicken and fennel. Cook for about 2 minutes, stirring occasionally until warmed through.

tip Fennel resembles celery, but with lacy leaves. Remove the celery-like stalks and set aside for another use. For the bulb, halve it lengthwise and use a paring knife to cut the core out of the bottom of the bulb on each side. From there, thinly slice.

PER SERVING (2 cups) Calories: 247; Total Fat: 14g; Saturated Fat: 2g; Cholesterol: 76mg; Carbohydrates: 5g; Fiber: 2g; Protein: 26g; Sodium: 513mg

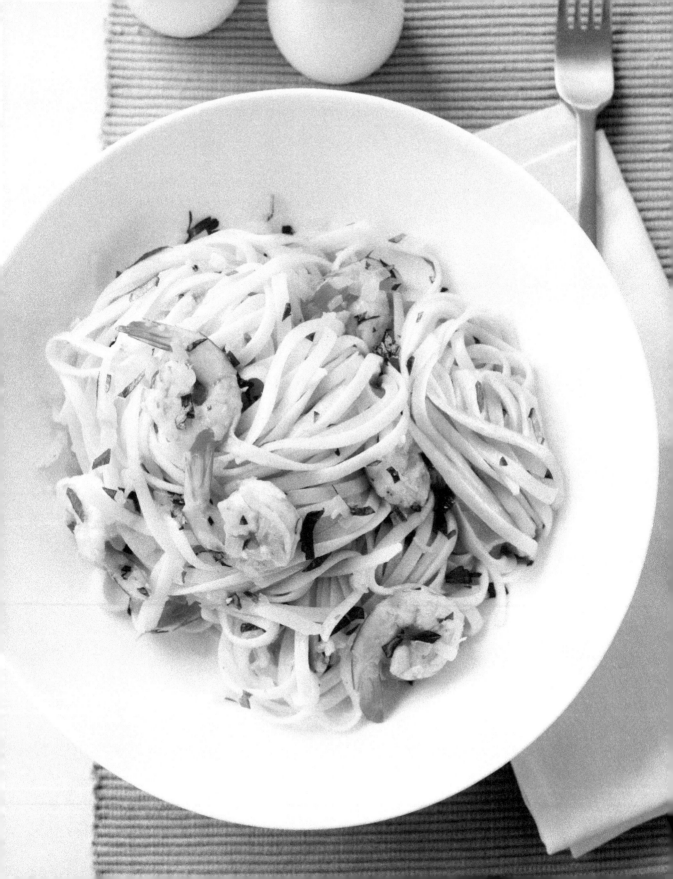

SEVEN

Fish & Shellfish

Shrimp *and* Pea Salad

ALKALINE **GLUTEN-FREE LOW-CARB**

Serves 4
Prep: 10 minutes

This fresh shrimp salad is refreshing, quick, and easy. It's a great summer dinner, or perfect for a light luncheon. Use the freshest shrimp you can find or thaw flash-frozen shrimp. What makes this salad delicious is the simplicity of the ingredients and their light, fresh flavors. The trick is to let the ingredients speak for themselves without overcomplicating them.

2 cups fresh peas
12 ounces cooked baby shrimp, chilled
¼ cup Greek Yogurt "Mayonnaise" (page 138)
¼ cup chopped fresh basil
2 tablespoons chopped fresh dill
½ teaspoon grated lemon zest
½ teaspoon sea salt
4 crisp lettuce leaves

1. In a large bowl, mix the peas and shrimp.

2. In a small bowl, whisk together the mayonnaise, basil, dill, lemon zest, and salt.

3. Toss the dressing with the salad.

4. Serve the salad in the lettuce leaves.

tip The most flavorful peas are those you have freshly shelled. Head to your local farmers' market in the spring to find tasty, tender peas.

PER SERVING (1 cup) Calories: 173; Total Fat: 2g; Saturated Fat: <1g; Cholesterol: 180mg; Carbohydrates: 14g; Fiber: 4g; Protein: 25g; Sodium: 850mg

Shrimp Tacos

ALKALINE   GLUTEN-FREE   LOW-CARB

Serves 4
Prep: 10 minutes
Cook: 15 minutes

You don't need to marinate shrimp long to infuse them with flavor—about five minutes is all it takes because of their delicate flesh. These shrimp tacos are perfect for Taco Tuesday because they are so quick and easy to make, and they are loaded with flavor.

4 corn tortillas

¼ cup extra-virgin olive oil, plus 2 tablespoons

2 tablespoons Vegetable Broth (page 134)

1 teaspoon ground cumin

1 teaspoon ground coriander

½ teaspoon sea salt

Zest of 1 lime

12 ounces jumbo shrimp, peeled, deveined, and tails removed

¼ cup chopped fresh cilantro

1. Preheat the oven to 325°F.

2. Wrap the tortillas in aluminum foil and place them in the oven to warm for about 15 minutes.

3. In a large bowl, whisk ¼ cup of oil, the broth, cumin, coriander, salt, and lime zest.

4. Stir in the shrimp. Let them marinate for 5 minutes.

5. In a 12-inch nonstick sauté pan or skillet over medium-high heat, heat the remaining 2 tablespoons of oil until it shimmers.

6. Remove the shrimp from the marinade and add them to the hot pan. Cook for about 4 minutes, stirring occasionally until the shrimp are opaque.

7. Serve the shrimp on the hot tortillas, sprinkled with the cilantro.

tip Add a dollop of sour cream (about 1 tablespoon) to each taco.

PER SERVING (1 tortilla and 3 ounces shrimp)
Calories: 217; Total Fat: 9g; Saturated Fat: 2g; Cholesterol: 179mg; Carbohydrates: 12g; Fiber: 2g; Protein: 21g; Sodium: 1,236mg

Shrimp Fried Rice

ALKALINE **GLUTEN-FREE** LOW-FODMAP

Serves 4
Prep: 10 minutes
Cook: 7 minutes

Craving Chinese take-out? Make a quick and easy fried rice to satisfy those cravings—your stomach will thank you. This tasty fried rice is ready in less than 20 minutes, and it's loaded with delicious and savory flavors.

2 tablespoons extra-virgin olive oil

6 ounces medium shrimp, peeled, deveined, and tails removed

2 carrots, peeled and cut into ¼-inch dice

2 teaspoons grated fresh ginger

3 cups cooked brown rice, hot

1 cup peas, fresh or frozen and thawed

¼ cup Easy Ginger Stir-Fry Sauce (page 141)

2 tablespoons chopped fresh cilantro

1. In a 12-inch nonstick sauté pan or skillet over medium-high heat, heat the oil until it shimmers.

2. Add the shrimp, carrots, and ginger. Cook for about 4 minutes, stirring occasionally until the vegetables are soft and the shrimp are opaque and cooked.

3. Stir in the rice, peas, and stir-fry sauce. Cook for 2 minutes, stirring constantly.

4. Remove from the heat and stir in the cilantro.

tip If you don't want to take the time to devein shrimp, buy frozen tail-off deveined shrimp at the grocery store. To thaw them quickly, place them in a colander under cold running water. They will thaw in less than 10 minutes.

PER SERVING (1½ cups) Calories: 417; Total Fat: 8g; Saturated Fat: 1g; Cholesterol: 90mg; Carbohydrates: 66g; Fiber: 4g; Protein: 18g; Sodium: 809mg

Honey *and* Cinnamon Glazed Shrimp

ALKALINE **GLUTEN-FREE** PALEO

Serves 4
Prep: 10 minutes
Cook: 5 minutes

Honey and cinnamon are perfect complements to the sweet succulence of shrimp. You can use either an indoor or outdoor grill—I make this on my George Foreman grill and it cooks twice as quickly. Grilling caramelizes the glaze on the outside of the shrimp in the most satisfying manner. Serve with hot rice or a side salad.

2 tablespoons honey
2 tablespoons Poultry Broth (page 132)
1 teaspoon Dijon mustard
1 teaspoon ground cinnamon
½ teaspoon grated orange zest
12 ounces jumbo shrimp, peeled
    and deveined

1. Heat the grill or a grill pan to medium-high heat.

2. In a medium bowl, whisk together the honey, broth, mustard, cinnamon, and orange zest.

3. Add the shrimp and toss to coat.

4. Grill the shrimp for about 5 minutes until opaque and cooked.

tip   To devein a shrimp, hold it under cold water and use the tip of a sharp knife to slice along the back above the vein, then remove the vein with the tip of the knife.

PER SERVING (3 ounces) Calories: 136; Total Fat: 2g; Saturated Fat: 0g; Cholesterol: 179mg; Carbohydrates: 11g; Fiber: 0g; Protein: 20g; Sodium: 224mg

Shrimp *and* Grits

Serves 4
Prep: 10 minutes
Cook: 15 minutes

You've probably been told to never mix seafood and cheese. Trust me, make an exception for shrimp and grits. Cheesy grits are the perfect foil for the shrimp; the two flavors blend well together for a simple yet special meal.

12 ounces medium shrimp, peeled and deveined
1 tablespoon extra-virgin olive oil
1 teaspoon sea salt, divided
4 cups Poultry Broth (page 132)
1 cup quick cooking grits
¼ cup grated fat-free Cheddar cheese

1. Heat the grill or a grill pan to medium-high heat.

2. Brush the shrimp with the oil and sprinkle with $1/2$ teaspoon of salt.

3. Grill the shrimp for about 4 minutes.

4. Meanwhile, in a medium saucepan over high heat, bring the broth and remaining $1/2$ teaspoon of salt to a boil.

5. Stir in the grits. Return to a boil, stirring constantly. Reduce the heat to medium-low and simmer for 4 minutes, stirring frequently.

6. Stir in the cheese. Cook for about 2 minutes, stirring constantly until the cheese melts.

7. Serve the grits topped with the shrimp.

tip Make the grits a bit creamier by stirring in 1 tablespoon unsalted butter and 1 tablespoon heavy (whipping) cream when you add the Cheddar cheese.

PER SERVING (3 ounces shrimp and ½ cup grits)
Calories: 238; Total Fat: 9g; Saturated Fat: 3g; Cholesterol: 187mg; Carbohydrates: 14g; Fiber: 2g; Protein: 25g; Sodium: 947mg

Pan-Seared Sea Scallops *with* Orange-Ginger Glaze

GLUTEN-FREE LOW-FODMAP PALEO

Serves 4
Prep: 10 minutes
Cook: 9 minutes

Sea scallops are the large scallops you'll find in the fresh seafood department of the grocery store. They are low in fat but have a delicate, sweet flavor that works well with the glaze in this recipe. Serve with rice or on a bed of greens.

1 pound sea scallops
½ teaspoon sea salt
2 tablespoons extra-virgin olive oil
¼ cup Vegetable Broth (page 134)
2 tablespoons honey
1 tablespoon grated fresh ginger
1 teaspoon grated orange zest

1. Season the scallops with the salt.

2. In a 12-inch nonstick sauté pan or skillet over medium-high heat, heat the oil until it shimmers.

3. Add the scallops. Cook for about 3 minutes per side until browned on both sides. Transfer to a plate and loosely tent with aluminum foil. Return the pan to the heat.

4. In a small bowl, whisk together the broth, honey, ginger, and orange zest. Add the glaze to the hot pan and bring to a simmer. Simmer for about 1 minute, stirring until thick and syrupy.

5. Return the scallops to the pan and toss to coat.

tip Sea scallops have a tough tendon on the side you need to remove. Insert the tip of a sharp knife underneath the tendon to separate it from the tender scallop.

PER SERVING (4 ounces scallops) Calories: 199; Total Fat: 8g; Saturated Fat: 1g; Cholesterol: 37mg; Carbohydrates: 13g; Fiber: 0g; Protein: 20g; Sodium: 442mg

Fish Fry

Serves 4
Prep: 10 minutes
Cook: 11 minutes

No need to forgo the Friday night fish fry. This version uses very little fat but still yields crispy, satisfying fish. Serve it with a side of Sweet Potato Oven "Fries" (page 54), Creamy Coleslaw (page 65), and some Buttermilk Ranch Dressing (page 137) in place of tartar sauce for a tasty dinner that doesn't taste like you're sacrificing anything.

1 egg, beaten
¼ cup low-fat buttermilk
1 cup all-purpose flour
1 teaspoon sea salt
1 teaspoon dried dill
12 ounces cod, cut into ½-inch pieces
2 tablespoons extra-virgin olive oil

1. In a shallow dish, whisk the egg and buttermilk together.

2. In another shallow dish, mix the flour, salt, and dill.

3. Dip the cod in the seasoned flour. Tap away any excess.

4. Dip it in the egg mixture and back in the flour mixture.

5. In a large nonstick sauté pan or skillet over medium-high heat, heat the oil until it shimmers.

6. Add the coated fish. Cook for about 5 minutes per side until golden on each side.

tip You can replace the cod with any local white fish, depending on what's available in your region.

PER SERVING (3 ounces fish) Calories: 286; Total Fat: 9g; Saturated Fat: 2g; Cholesterol: 88mg; Carbohydrates: 25g; Fiber: <1g; Protein: 25g; Sodium: 666mg

Fish Sticks *with* Tartar Sauce

Serves 4
Prep: 10 minutes
Cook: 12 minutes

Using panko bread crumbs yields a super-crispy exterior that makes these fish sticks crunchy and delicious. Baking reduces fat and only takes about 10 minutes. Serve these with Baked Potato Chips (page 53) or a simple salad for a quick and easy meal.

FOR THE FISH STICKS
Nonstick cooking spray
1 cup panko bread crumbs
1 teaspoon sea salt
1 teaspoon dried thyme
12 ounces cod, cut into ½-inch pieces
2 eggs, beaten

FOR THE TARTAR SAUCE
½ cup nonfat plain Greek-style yogurt
2 tablespoons chopped fresh dill
1 teaspoon Dijon mustard
1 teaspoon lemon zest

TO MAKE THE FISH STICKS

1. Preheat the oven to 400°F.

2. Spray a baking sheet with nonstick cooking spray.

3. In a shallow dish, mix the bread crumbs, salt, and thyme.

4. Dip the cod in the beaten eggs and into the bread crumb mixture. Place on the prepared sheet.

5. Bake for about 12 minutes until golden and the fish is cooked.

TO MAKE THE TARTAR SAUCE

In a small bowl, stir together the yogurt, dill, mustard, and lemon zest. Refrigerate until serving.

tip This recipe also works well with salmon, although the fat content is a little higher, but you can use whatever fish is available in your region.

PER SERVING (3 ounces fish with 2 tablespoons tartar sauce) Calories: 303; Total Fat: 9g; Saturated Fat: 2g; Cholesterol: 89mg; Carbohydrates: 27g; Fiber: 1g; Protein: 26g; Sodium: 597mg

Tarragon Baked Cod

GLUTEN-FREE **LOW-CARB** LOW-FODMAP PALEO

Serves 4
Prep: 5 minutes
Cook: 20 minutes

This simple baked fish makes the most of the few ingredients it uses. The highlight is on simple, delicious flavors. Choose the freshest cod you can find. It should be pearly white and have a briny (but not fishy) aroma when you sniff it.

Nonstick cooking spray
4 (3-ounce) skinless cod fillets
1 tablespoon extra-virgin olive oil
1 teaspoon dried tarragon
½ teaspoon sea salt
½ teaspoon grated lemon zest

1. Preheat the oven to 400°F.

2. Spray a baking sheet with nonstick cooking spray.

3. Place the cod on the prepared sheet. Brush each piece with oil.

4. In a small bowl, mix the tarragon, salt, and lemon zest. Sprinkle this onto the fish.

5. Bake for 15 to 20 minutes until the fish is opaque.

tip A little black pepper zips up these ingredients. Try adding ⅛ teaspoon freshly ground black pepper (if you tolerate it well) to the herb and salt mixture.

PER SERVING (3 ounces) Calories: 120; Total Fat: 4g; Saturated Fat: <1g; Cholesterol: 47mg; Carbohydrates: <1g; Fiber: 0g; Protein: 20g; Sodium: 300mg

Cod with Spinach Pesto

ALKALINE **GLUTEN-FREE LOW-CARB** PALEO

Serves 4
Prep: 10 minutes
Cook: 10 minutes

Cod is an affordable fish that's really easy to prepare and cook. Spinach pesto adds a beautiful bright green color to the delicate white fish and also brings plenty of flavor. Serve it with sautéed zucchini or a simple salad for a complete, nutritious, GERD-friendly meal.

4 (3-ounce) cod fillets
½ teaspoon sea salt
1 tablespoon extra-virgin olive oil
1 cup Spinach Pesto (page 139)

1. Season the fish fillets with salt.

2. In a 12-inch nonstick sauté pan or skillet over medium-high heat, heat the olive oil until it shimmers.

3. Add the fish. Cook for about 4 minutes per side until opaque.

4. Serve the fish topped with the pesto.

PER SERVING (3 ounces fish with 4 tablespoons pesto) Calories: 158; Total Fat: 7g; Saturated Fat: 1g; Cholesterol: 48mg; Carbohydrates: <1g; Fiber: 0g; Protein: 20g; Sodium: 417mg

White Fish *with* Mustard Cream Sauce

GLUTEN-FREE LOW-CARB

Serves 4
Prep: 10 minutes
Cook: 12 minutes

A creamy mustard and herb sauce complements this white fish, bringing richness to the dish. You can use any white fish that's available in your region. Halibut is one of my favorites, but I live pretty close to Alaska on the West Coast, so there's a lot of it around here. Flounder, snapper, and cod are other good choices.

4 (3-ounce) skinless halibut fillets
½ teaspoon sea salt
1 tablespoon unsalted butter
1 cup Vegetable Broth (page 134)
1 tablespoon Dijon mustard
1 tablespoon chopped fresh dill
Zest of 1 lemon
2 tablespoons heavy (whipping) cream

1. Season the fish fillets with the salt.

2. In a 12-inch nonstick sauté pan or skillet over medium-high heat, melt the butter until it bubbles.

3. Add the fish. Cook for about 3 minutes per side until opaque. Remove from the pan and tent loosely with aluminum foil. Return the pan to the heat.

4. In a small bowl, whisk together the broth, mustard, dill, and lemon zest. Add this to the hot pan. Cook 3 to 5 minutes, stirring until the liquid has reduced by half.

5. Whisk in the heavy cream.

6. Return the fish to the pan and turn to coat.

tip You'll need to check any fish you use for pin bones. Use a small pair of needlenose pliers to remove them quickly and easily.

PER SERVING (3 ounces) Calories: 155;
Total Fat: 7g; Saturated Fat: 4g; Cholesterol: 65mg;
Carbohydrates: 1g; Fiber: 0g; Protein: 21g;
Sodium: 559mg

Herb and Sour Cream Baked Halibut

Serves 4
Prep: 10 minutes
Cook: 20 minutes

One of the things I really like about preparing fish is how quickly it cooks. It doesn't take much time on the heat for the flesh to turn opaque and flake, although if you're not careful it's easy to overcook, for the same reason. This recipe helps adjust for overcooking because the sour cream topping helps keep it moist.

4 (3-ounce) skinless halibut fillets
½ teaspoon sea salt
1 cup fat-free sour cream
1 tablespoon chopped fresh dill
1 tablespoon chopped fresh parsley
1 teaspoon dried thyme

1. Preheat the oven to 350°F.

2. Line a rimmed baking sheet with parchment paper. Place the halibut fillets on the prepared sheet and sprinkle with the salt.

3. In a small bowl, mix the sour cream, dill, parsley, and thyme. Spread the mixture on the halibut.

4. Bake for about 20 minutes until the halibut flakes easily with a fork.

tip If halibut isn't readily available, try sole, flounder, cod, or another white fish available in your region.

PER SERVING (3 ounces) Calories: 152;
Total Fat: <1g; Saturated Fat: 0g; Cholesterol: 53mg;
Carbohydrates: 11g; Fiber: 0g; Protein: 22g;
Sodium: 353mg

Orange-Tarragon Salmon

GLUTEN-FREE LOW-CARB PALEO

Serves 4
Prep: 5 minutes
Cook: 20 minutes

Salmon is plentiful here in the Pacific Northwest where I live, so it frequently appears on the dinner table. While it's a fattier fish than white fish, it's chock-full of healthy anti-inflammatory omega-3 fatty acids. Here, delicate tarragon and tasty orange give it the perfect flavor boost.

4 (3-ounce) salmon fillets
1 tablespoon extra-virgin olive oil
1 tablespoon honey
2 tablespoons chopped fresh tarragon
1 teaspoon grated orange zest
½ teaspoon sea salt

1. Preheat the oven to 350°F.

2. Line a rimmed baking sheet with parchment paper. Place the salmon on the prepared sheet.

3. In a small bowl, whisk the oil and honey together. Brush this on the salmon.

4. In another small bowl, mix the tarragon, orange zest, and salt. Sprinkle this mixture on the salmon.

5. Bake for about 20 minutes until the salmon flakes easily with a fork.

tip   If you need this to be low-FODMAP, eliminate the honey.

PER SERVING (3 ounces) Calories: 161; Total Fat: 9g; Saturated Fat: 1g; Cholesterol: 38mg; Carbohydrates: 5g; Fiber: 0g; Protein: 17g; Sodium: 272mg

Cheesy Tuna Casserole

Serves 4
Prep: 10 minutes
Cook: 20 minutes

Tuna casserole is classic comfort food for many, and my family is no exception. This version again breaks the "rule" many foodies have against cheese and fish in the same dish, but the cheese adds richness and flavor here that makes this classic comfort food at its finest.

2 cups Mushroom Gravy (page 143)

8 ounces rotini pasta, cooked according to package instructions and drained

1 cup peas, fresh or frozen and thawed

1 (5-ounce) can water-packed tuna, drained and flaked

Zest of 1 lemon

¼ cup grated fat-free sharp Cheddar cheese

¼ cup panko bread crumbs

1 tablespoon unsalted butter, melted

1. Preheat the oven to 350°F.

2. In a large bowl, mix the gravy, pasta, peas, tuna, and lemon zest.

3. Spoon the mixture evenly into four (6- to 8-ounce) ramekins.

4. In a small bowl, combine the Cheddar cheese, bread crumbs, and butter. Sprinkle on top of the ramekins.

5. Bake for about 20 minutes until the casserole is bubbly and the topping is browned.

tip Tuna often has high levels of mercury; if you can find it, use safe-caught tuna, such as Safe Catch, which is available online at Thrive Market.

PER SERVING (6 ounces) Calories: 343; Total Fat: 10g; Saturated Fat: 4g; Cholesterol: 61mg; Carbohydrates: 40g; Fiber: 2g; Protein: 23g; Sodium: 490mg

Shrimp Linguine

Serves 4
Prep: 10 minutes
Cook: 10 minutes

This linguine's light sauce and succulent, flavorful shrimp create a satisfying GERD-friendly dinner. Serve it with a nice crusty bread on the side, as well as a simple salad for a delicious weeknight meal.

2 tablespoons extra-virgin olive oil

1 pound medium shrimp, peeled and deveined

2 cups Poultry Broth (page 132)

Zest of 1 lemon

½ teaspoon sea salt

1 tablespoon heavy (whipping) cream

1 tablespoon chopped fresh basil

8 ounces linguine, cooked according to package directions and drained

1. In a large sauté pan or skillet over medium-high heat, heat the oil until it shimmers.

2. Add the shrimp. Cook for about 4 minutes, stirring occasionally until opaque.

3. Stir in the broth, lemon zest, and salt. Simmer for 5 minutes, stirring occasionally.

4. Stir in the heavy cream and basil. Spoon over the hot pasta.

tip Sprinkle 1 tablespoon grated Parmesan cheese (if you tolerate it well) over each portion.

PER SERVING (1 cup pasta with ½ cup sauce) Calories: 213; Total Fat: 3g; Saturated Fat: 1g; Cholesterol: 47mg; Carbohydrates: 36g; Fiber: 0g; Protein: 9g; Sodium: 493mg

Smoked Salmon Pasta

Serves 4
Prep: 10 minutes
Cook: 6 minutes

You can find smoked salmon in the fish department of most grocery stores, and it's widely available online. The deep, rich, smoky flavor is strong, so a little goes a very long way in this tasty and easy-to-make pasta.

2 cups Poultry Broth (page 132)

1 cup peas, fresh or frozen and thawed

1 teaspoon dried thyme

Zest of 1 orange

2 tablespoons heavy (whipping) cream

8 ounces penne pasta, cooked according to package directions and drained

4 ounces smoked salmon, roughly chopped

1. In a medium pot over medium-high heat, simmer the broth for about 4 minutes, or until it has reduced by about one-fourth.

2. Add the peas, thyme, and orange zest. Simmer for 1 minute more.

3. Stir in the heavy cream. Cook for 1 minute, stirring.

4. Add the pasta and salmon. Toss to coat and serve immediately.

tip This dish is great with fresh crab, too. Replace the salmon with 6 ounces fresh lump crabmeat.

PER SERVING (1 cup pasta with ½ cup sauce)
Calories: 272; Total Fat: 6g; Saturated Fat: 2g; Cholesterol: 58mg; Carbohydrates: 37g; Fiber: 2g; Protein: 16g; Sodium: 622mg

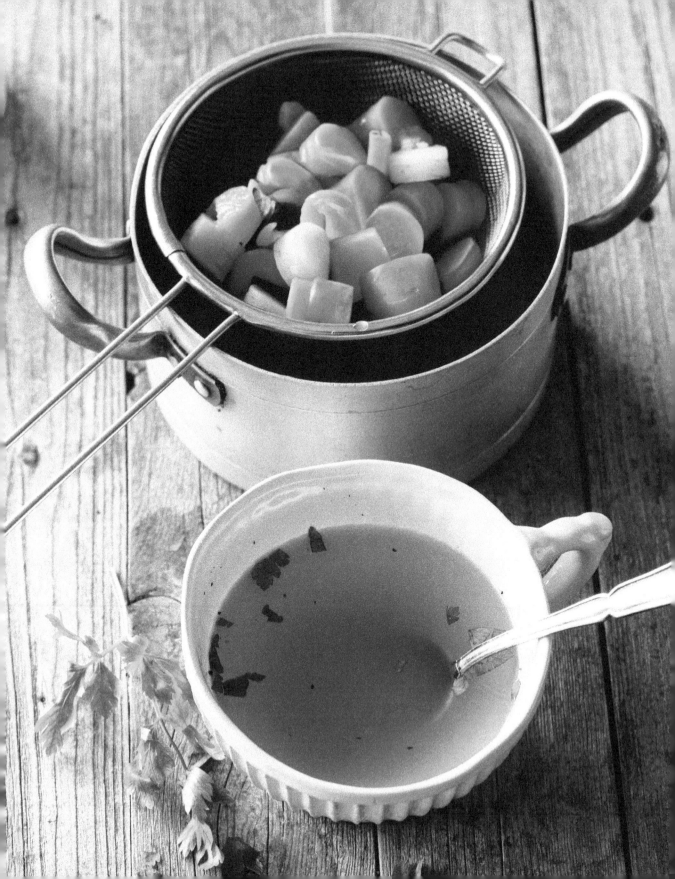

EIGHT

Broths, Sauces & Condiments

Poultry Broth

ALKALINE **GLUTEN-FREE** **LOW-CARB** LOW-FODMAP PALEO

Makes 3 to 5 quarts
Prep: 10 minutes
Cook: 2 to 24 hours

While most other recipes in this book take 30 minutes or less, the broth recipes are a little different. Broth requires a long simmering time to extract the flavors from its ingredients, so a long, slow-simmered broth is essential for building great flavor in foods. It serves as the flavor base for many of the recipes in this cookbook. Fortunately, active time is only about 15 minutes.

3 pounds chicken, turkey, or duck parts
    such as necks, backs, or wings
3 carrots, roughly chopped
3 celery stalks, roughly chopped
2 fresh rosemary sprigs
2 fresh thyme sprigs
1 teaspoon sea salt

1. In a large pot, or in a 6-quart slow cooker, combine the poultry pieces, carrots, celery, rosemary, thyme, and salt. Cover with enough cold water so the pot is about three-fourths full.

2. If using a slow cooker, cover and cook for 12 to 24 hours on low. If cooking on the stove top, place the pot over medium-low heat and bring to a simmer. Reduce the heat to low and simmer for 2 to 4 hours. The longer you simmer, the more flavorful the broth will be. Turn off the heat and let the broth cool slightly. Strain out and discard the solids.

3. Refrigerate the broth, covered, overnight. The fat will rise to the top and solidify. Skim away and discard the fat. Freeze the broth in 1- or 2-cup portions for up to 12 months, or refrigerate for up to 5 days and use as needed.

tip Freeze bones from poultry meals and vegetable trimmings like carrot peels and celery tops in a zip-top bag in the freezer. Use these scraps to make the broth. It's a great, economical, nonwasteful way to make healthy food.

PER SERVING (1 cup) Calories: 38; Total Fat: 0g; Saturated Fat: 0g; Cholesterol: 0mg; Carbohydrates: <1g; Fiber: 0g; Protein: 5g; Sodium: 70mg

Vegetable Broth

ALKALINE **GLUTEN-FREE** **LOW-CARB** LOW-FODMAP PALEO VEGAN

Makes 3 to 5 quarts
Prep: 10 minutes
Cook: 1 to 12 hours

You don't need animal products to make a flavorful broth. You can make a delicious broth from vegetables. Freeze vegetable scraps from your cooking, such as carrot greens, fennel fronds and tops, mushroom stems, and celery tops and leaves, in a large zip-top bag and use these to make broth. Vegetables don't take as long to give up their flavors for a flavorful broth—the best flavors come in about 2 to 3 hours of simmering (or 8 to 12 hours in a slow cooker).

4 carrots, roughly chopped
4 celery stalks, roughly chopped
1 fennel bulb, roughly chopped
8 ounces mushrooms
¼ cup fresh parsley leaves
2 fresh rosemary sprigs
2 fresh thyme sprigs
1 teaspoon sea salt

1. In a large pot, or in a 6-quart slow cooker, combine the carrots, celery, fennel, mushrooms, parsley, rosemary, thyme, and salt. Cover with enough cold water so the pot is about three-fourths full.

2. If using a slow cooker, cover and cook for 8 to 12 hours on low. If cooking on the stove top, place the pot over medium-low heat and bring to a simmer. Reduce the heat to low and simmer for 1 to 3 hours. Longer simmering times yield a more flavorful broth. Turn off the heat and let the broth cool slightly. Strain out and discard the solids.

3. Freeze the broth in 1- or 2-cup portions for up to 12 months, or refrigerate for up to 5 days and use as needed.

tip If saving vegetable scraps for broth, avoid strongly flavored vegetables such as cauliflower, cabbage, kale, spinach, or broccoli. These will impart "off" flavors. Focus on root vegetables (except onions) and mushrooms.

PER SERVING (1 cup) Calories: 38; Total Fat: 0g; Saturated Fat: 0g; Cholesterol: 0mg; Carbohydrates: <1g; Fiber: 0g; Protein: 5g; Sodium: 70mg

Mushroom Broth

ALKALINE **GLUTEN-FREE** **LOW-CARB** LOW-FODMAP PALEO VEGAN

Makes 6 cups
Prep: 5 minutes
Cook: 5 minutes
Steep: 2 to 4 hours

Dried mushrooms add deep savory, earthy flavors to this broth. This recipe uses Vegetable Broth (page 134) as the base, and mushrooms infuse the flavor required for many soups and sauces in this cookbook. In my cooking, I find it adds a depth of flavor I can't get with regular broth.

6 cups Vegetable Broth (page 134)
2 ounces dried porcini mushrooms

1. In a medium saucepan over high heat, bring the broth to a boil.

2. Stir in the dried mushrooms and remove the pan from the heat. Cover and let the mushrooms steep in the broth for 2 to 4 hours. Strain the broth and discard the mushrooms.

3. Freeze the broth in 1- or 2-cup portions for up to 12 months, or refrigerate for up to 5 days and use as needed.

tip Dried porcini mushrooms have the best flavor for this recipe, but if you can't find them, use dried shiitake or dried cremini mushrooms instead. You can find dried mushrooms in the produce section of your local grocery store.

PER SERVING (1 cup) Calories: 38; Total Fat: 0g; Saturated Fat: 0g; Cholesterol: 0mg; Carbohydrates: <1g; Fiber: 0g; Protein: 5g; Sodium: 70mg

Low-Fat White Sauce

GLUTEN-FREE **LOW-CARB** VEGETARIAN

Makes 3 cups
Prep: 5 minutes
Cook: 6 minutes

This low-fat white sauce is simple and delicious, and it only takes a few minutes to make. It serves as a great base for many of the recipes in this cookbook. The trick is to whisk it constantly while it heats to keep the dairy from burning and allow the ingredients to incorporate completely.

2 tablespoons unsalted butter
3 tablespoons gluten-free flour
2 cups Vegetable Broth (page 134)
1 cup skim milk
Pinch ground nutmeg
¼ teaspoon sea salt

1. In a saucepan over medium-high heat, melt the butter until it bubbles.

2. Whisk in the flour and cook for 2 minutes, whisking constantly.

3. Whisk in the broth and milk. Cook for about 3 minutes, whisking constantly until thickened.

4. Whisk in the nutmeg and salt.

tip Add ¼ cup freshly grated Parmesan cheese (if you tolerate it well) to pump up the flavor.

PER SERVING (¼ cup) Calories: 38; Total Fat: 2g; Saturated Fat: 2g; Cholesterol: 6mg; Carbohydrates: 3g; Fiber: 0g; Protein: 2g; Sodium: 513mg

Buttermilk Ranch Dressing

GLUTEN-FREE LOW-CARB VEGETARIAN

Makes 1 cup
Prep: 5 minutes

This low-fat ranch dressing and dip is perfect to top a salad, and is delicious as a burger spread or as a veggie or chip dip. It keeps in the refrigerator for about three days, so it's best to make it fresh when you need it. It's so quick and easy, you'll find yourself whipping up a batch whenever you long for that tangy flavor.

¾ cup low-fat buttermilk
¼ cup nonfat plain Greek-style yogurt
1 tablespoon chopped fresh dill
1 tablespoon chopped fresh thyme
1 tablespoon chopped fresh rosemary
1 tablespoon chopped fresh parsley
½ teaspoon grated lemon zest
½ teaspoon sea salt

In a small bowl, whisk together the buttermilk, yogurt, dill, thyme, rosemary, parsley, lemon zest, and salt. Refrigerate for about 30 minutes to blend the flavors.

tip Add ⅛ teaspoon freshly ground black pepper (if you tolerate it well) to pump up the flavor.

PER SERVING (2 tablespoons) Calories: 17; Total Fat: <1g; Saturated Fat: 0g; Cholesterol: 1mg; Carbohydrates: 2g; Fiber: 0g; Protein: 1g; Sodium: 74mg

Greek Yogurt "Mayonnaise"

GLUTEN-FREE   LOW-CARB   VEGETARIAN

Makes 1 cup
Prep: 5 minutes
Chill: 30 minutes

You can always opt to buy fat-free mayonnaise, but commercially prepared fat-free mayo has lots of chemical ingredients. This fresh, easy version gives you lots of flavor without the fat, and it makes a great base for salad dressings, dips, and spreads for sandwiches or burgers. It will keep refrigerated for about five days.

1 cup nonfat plain Greek-style yogurt
1 teaspoon Dijon mustard
Zest of 1 lemon
½ teaspoon sea salt

In a small bowl, whisk together the yogurt, mustard, lemon zest, and salt. Refrigerate for 30 minutes to blend the flavors.

tip   Add ⅛ teaspoon freshly ground black pepper (if you tolerate it well) to pump up the flavor.

PER SERVING (2 tablespoons) Calories: 18; Total Fat: <1g; Saturated Fat: 0g; Cholesterol: 1mg; Carbohydrates: 2g; Fiber: 0g; Protein: 2g; Sodium: 74mg

Spinach Pesto

ALKALINE **GLUTEN-FREE** **LOW-CARB** VEGETARIAN

Makes 1 cup
Prep: 5 minutes

You'll really love the bright flavors in this pesto, which whips up quickly in a blender or food processor. It's a tasty addition to pasta or egg dishes, and a great topping for low-fat meats. It keeps in the refrigerator for up to five days. You can also freeze tablespoon-size servings in an ice cube tray and pop out just what you need for instant flavor.

1 cup fresh baby spinach
½ cup fresh basil leaves
½ cup grated fat-free Parmesan cheese
¼ cup extra-virgin olive oil
Zest of 1 lemon
½ teaspoon sea salt

In a blender or food processor, combine the spinach, basil, Parmesan cheese, oil, lemon zest, and salt. Pulse for about 20 (1-second) pulses until all the ingredients are ground.

tip Add 2 tablespoons pine nuts for a richer, more traditional flavor.

PER SERVING (1 tablespoon) Calories: 39; Total Fat: 3g; Saturated Fat: <1g; Cholesterol: 1mg; Carbohydrates: <1g; Fiber: 0g; Protein: 1g; Sodium: 117mg

Umami Burger Sauce

GLUTEN-FREE LOW-CARB VEGETARIAN

Makes ½ cup
Prep: 5 minutes

This sweet and savory burger sauce is a natural for topping burgers or sandwiches, but it's also tasty as a dip for fries, chips, veggies, or even fat-free pretzels. It will keep in the refrigerator for three to five days, but it's so easy to make you can whip up a batch anytime. It's the go-to burger topper in my house.

½ cup Greek Yogurt "Mayonnaise" (page 138)
1 tablespoon gluten-free soy sauce
1 tablespoon packed brown sugar
1 tablespoon chopped fresh thyme

In a small bowl, whisk together the mayonnaise, soy sauce, brown sugar, and thyme until the sugar has completely dissolved.

tip Add a pinch of freshly ground black pepper (if you tolerate it well).

PER SERVING (2 tablespoons) Calories: 15; Total Fat: <1g; Saturated Fat: 0g; Cholesterol: 0mg; Carbohydrates: 3g; Fiber: 0g; Protein: 1g; Sodium: 100mg

Easy Ginger Stir-Fry Sauce

GLUTEN-FREE   LOW-CARB   VEGAN

Makes 1 cup
Prep: 5 minutes

This quick stir-fry sauce will keep in the refrigerator for up to five days, or you can freeze it in ice cube trays in tablespoon-size servings. Once frozen, pop out the cubes, and store them in a labeled zip-top bag. When you need some sauce, take out the needed number of cubes and add them to your recipe. How easy is that?

1 cup gluten-free soy sauce
2 tablespoons pure maple syrup
1 tablespoon grated fresh ginger
Zest of 1 lime
¼ teaspoon ground coriander

In a small bowl, whisk together the soy sauce, maple syrup, ginger, lime zest, and coriander.

tip   You can use 2 teaspoons ground ginger instead of fresh ginger.

PER SERVING (2 tablespoons) Calories: 35; Total Fat: <1g; Saturated Fat: 0g; Cholesterol: 0mg; Carbohydrates: 7g; Fiber: 0g; Protein: 2g; Sodium: 899mg

Honey Mustard Dipping Sauce

GLUTEN-FREE   LOW-CARB

Makes 1 cup
Prep: 5 minutes

Another quick sauce to whip up, this one is perfect as a salad dressing, and it's delicious as a dip for fish or chicken, or as a sauce to top meat, fish, and poultry. Refrigerate it, tightly sealed, for up to five days.

1 cup Greek Yogurt "Mayonnaise" (page 138)
2 tablespoons honey
1 tablespoon yellow mustard
Pinch sea salt

In a small bowl, whisk together the mayonnaise, honey, mustard, and salt.

tip   Whisk in ½ teaspoon grated orange zest for a light citrus flavor.

PER SERVING (2 tablespoons) Calories: 34; Total Fat: <1g; Saturated Fat: 0g; Cholesterol: 1mg; Carbohydrates: 7g; Fiber: 0g; Protein: 2g; Sodium: 66mg

Mushroom Gravy

GLUTEN-FREE LOW-CARB PALEO VEGAN

Makes 2 cups
Prep: 5 minutes
Cook: 7 minutes

Who said gravy is off-limits? This version is used as a flavor base in several recipes throughout this cookbook. Arrowroot powder thickens the gravy but keeps it gluten-free and paleo. If you can't find arrowroot powder, substitute cornstarch.

2 cups Mushroom Broth (page 135), divided
3 tablespoons arrowroot powder
1 teaspoon chopped fresh thyme
½ teaspoon sea salt

1. In a saucepan over medium-high heat, heat 1½ cups of broth until it simmers.

2. In a small bowl, whisk together the remaining ½ cup of broth, arrowroot powder, thyme, and salt. Whisk this into the simmering broth. Cook for about 2 minutes, stirring constantly until thickened.

tip Whisk in ⅛ teaspoon freshly ground black pepper (if you tolerate it well) to add flavor.

PER SERVING (¼ cup) Calories: 12; Total Fat: <1g; Saturated Fat: 0g; Cholesterol: 0mg; Carbohydrates: <1g; Fiber: 0g; Protein: 1g; Sodium: 135mg

Brown Sugar Peach Topping

ALKALINE **GLUTEN-FREE** VEGAN

Makes 1½ cups
Prep: 5 minutes
Cook: 5 minutes

This recipe uses canned peaches, which are much lower in acidity than fresh peaches. Select peaches canned in water, not syrup. This topping is delicious on pancakes or waffles, and is a tasty accompaniment to a low-fat dessert like fat-free frozen yogurt. This will keep in the refrigerator for up to five days or in the freezer for up to one year.

1 (15-ounce) can water-packed
   peaches, drained
¼ cup packed brown sugar
1 teaspoon ground cinnamon
¼ teaspoon ground nutmeg
¼ teaspoon ground ginger
Pinch sea salt

1. In a blender, purée the peaches. Transfer to a medium saucepan and place it over medium-high heat.

2. Stir in the brown sugar, cinnamon, nutmeg, ginger, and salt. Cook for about 5 minutes, stirring constantly until it simmers and the brown sugar dissolves. Serve warm or chilled.

tip Stir in 2 tablespoons finely chopped pecans for texture.

PER SERVING (¼ cup) Calories: 172; Total Fat: 1g; Saturated Fat: 0g; Cholesterol: 0mg; Carbohydrates: 41g; Fiber: 6g; Protein: 4g; Sodium: 41mg

French Fry Sauce

GLUTEN-FREE LOW-CARB

Makes 1 cup
Prep: 5 minutes

If you're looking for a sauce to dip your fries in, this is the one! It's also good on burgers or as a vegetable dip. It does contain a small amount of tomato sauce for flavor, but as long as you keep your portions at less than two tablespoons, this sauce shouldn't activate your acid reflux.

1 cup Greek Yogurt "Mayonnaise" (page 138)
1 tablespoon tomato sauce
1 teaspoon gluten-free soy sauce
1 teaspoon chopped fresh dill
¼ teaspoon fish sauce

In a small bowl, whisk together the mayonnaise, tomato sauce, soy sauce, dill, and fish sauce.

tip Want to make it vegetarian? Omit the fish sauce.

PER SERVING (2 tablespoons) Calories: 18; Total Fat: <1g; Saturated Fat: 0g; Cholesterol: 1mg; Carbohydrates: 3g; Fiber: 0g; Protein: 1g; Sodium: 148mg

Curry Mayonnaise

GLUTEN-FREE **LOW-CARB** VEGETARIAN

Makes 1 cup
Prep: 5 minutes

This is great on burgers, with fish or poultry, and as a dip for fries, chips, and veggies. It will keep refrigerated for three to five days, but it's so easy to whip up fresh that there's no need to make it ahead of time. The delicious curry adds a huge boost of flavor and aroma.

1 cup Greek Yogurt "Mayonnaise" (page 138)
1 teaspoon curry powder
½ teaspoon grated lime zest
¼ teaspoon sea salt

In a small bowl, whisk together the mayonnaise, curry powder, lime zest, and salt.

tip If making a nonvegetarian mayonnaise, add a dash of fish sauce to pump up the flavor—about ⅛ teaspoon.

PER SERVING (2 tablespoons) Calories: 18; Total Fat: <1g; Saturated Fat: 0g; Cholesterol: 1mg; Carbohydrates: 3g; Fiber: 0g; Protein: 1g; Sodium: 148mg

Creamy Avocado Coleslaw Dressing

ALKALINE **GLUTEN-FREE** **LOW-CARB** PALEO VEGETARIAN

Makes 1 cup
Prep: 5 minutes

Make this quick, easy dressing in the blender for coleslaw, or as a tasty ranch substitution for other salads. Because it lacks acid, this dressing does not store well, so plan on making only as much as you need.

1 avocado, peeled, halved, and pitted
¼ cup unsweetened almond milk
Zest of 1 lime
1 tablespoon grated fresh ginger
1 tablespoon honey
½ teaspoon sea salt
⅛ teaspoon freshly ground black
    pepper (optional)

In a blender, process the avocado, almond milk, lime zest, ginger, honey, salt, and pepper (if using) until smooth.

tip To make it vegan, replace the honey with one packet of stevia.

PER SERVING (2 tablespoons) Calories: 63;
Total Fat: 5g; Saturated Fat: 1g; Cholesterol: 0mg;
Carbohydrates: 5g; Fiber: 2g; Protein: <1g;
Sodium: 120mg

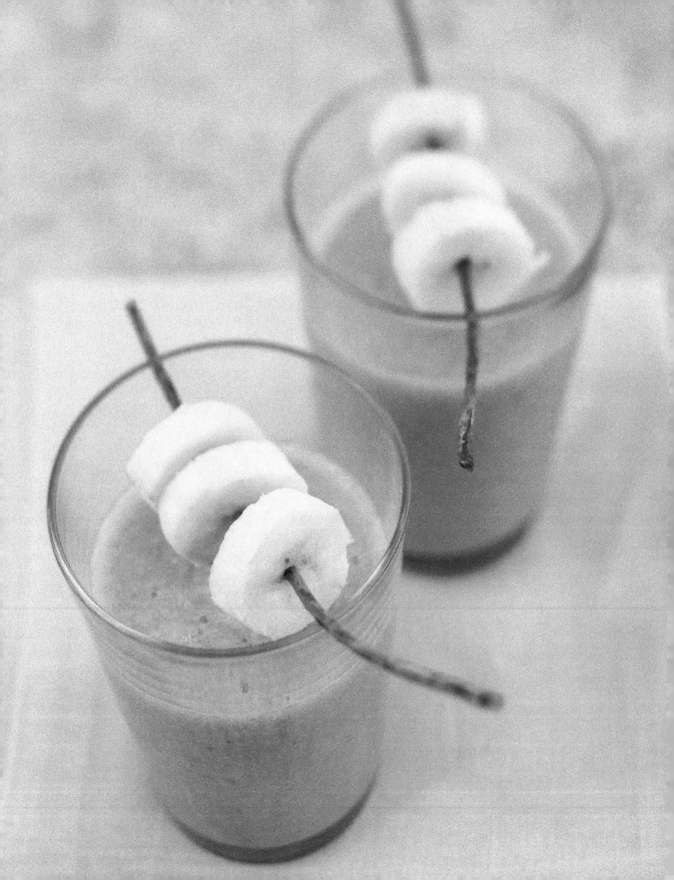

NINE

Snacks & Sweets

Caramel Corn

ALKALINE **GLUTEN-FREE** VEGETARIAN

Makes 5 servings
Prep: 5 minutes
Cook: 10 minutes

This sticky, gooey treat is a tasty way to enjoy popcorn, and it's easy and quick. It's a perfect snack for family movie night or game day. Be sure to keep portions strictly in check so you don't overfill your stomach.

¼ cup pure maple syrup
¼ cup packed dark brown sugar
1 tablespoon unsalted butter
⅛ teaspoon sea salt
Nonstick cooking spray
5 cups air-popped popcorn

1. In a medium saucepan over medium-high heat, cook the maple syrup, brown sugar, butter, and salt for 5 to 10 minutes, stirring constantly until the sugar has dissolved.

2. Coat a large bowl with nonstick cooking spray. Add the popcorn.

3. Pour in the caramel sauce and stir to coat. Serve warm.

tip If you don't have an air popper, use microwave popcorn, but use a low-fat variety.

PER SERVING (1 cup) Calories: 120; Total Fat: 3g; Saturated Fat: 2g; Cholesterol: 6mg; Carbohydrates: 24g; Fiber: 1g; Protein: 1g; Sodium: 79mg

Spiced Hot Cider

GLUTEN-FREE PALEO VEGAN

Makes 8 servings
Prep: 5 minutes
Cook: 20 minutes

This is a sweet treat by itself, or a great accompaniment to Caramel Corn (page 150) for a tasty snack. I like to make batches of spiced hot cider in the fall, especially for fall gatherings such as Thanksgiving. When I do, I make a big batch in my slow cooker and keep it on the warm setting for people to drink throughout the day.

8 cups apple cider
¼ cup pure maple syrup
8 whole allspice
4 whole cloves
3 cinnamon sticks
1 (1-inch) piece fresh ginger
Pinch ground nutmeg

1. In a large pot over medium heat, stir together the cider, maple syrup, allspice, cloves, cinnamon, ginger, and nutmeg.

2. Bring to a simmer. Cook for 20 minutes, stirring occasionally. Strain out the solids before serving.

tip Brown sugar is an inexpensive substitute for pure maple syrup. You can replace the syrup with ¼ cup packed dark brown sugar.

PER SERVING (1 cup) Calories: 142; Total Fat: <1g; Saturated Fat: 0g; Cholesterol: 0mg; Carbohydrates: 36g; Fiber: 0g; Protein: <1g; Sodium: 8mg

White Hot Chocolate

Serves 4
Prep: 5 minutes
Cook: 10 minutes

While the white chocolate in this has a fair amount of fat, small portion sizes will keep it from triggering acid reflux. This is a great treat if you crave hot chocolate—it gives you all the warmth and flavor without activating your acid reflux like chocolate does.

6 ounces white chocolate chips
4 cups skim milk
½ teaspoon alcohol-free vanilla extract
Pinch sea salt

1. In a medium saucepan over medium heat, stir together the white chocolate chips, milk, vanilla, and salt.

2. Bring to a simmer, stirring constantly, and cook for about 5 minutes, until the chocolate has melted.

tip Just as you would with your favorite hot chocolate, serve this one topped with mini marshmallows (but remember it won't be vegetarian).

PER SERVING (1 cup) Calories: 321; Total Fat: 14g; Saturated Fat: 8g; Cholesterol: 14mg; Carbohydrates: 37g; Fiber: 0g; Protein: 11; Sodium: 207mg

Fruit *and* Yogurt Parfaits

Makes 2 parfaits
Prep: 10 minutes

These tangy, slightly sweet parfaits are a perfect dessert. They are light and won't overfill you, but will leave you feeling satisfied. Because they are so quick to prepare, make them just before serving.

2 (6-ounce) containers nonfat plain
   Greek-style yogurt
2 tablespoons honey
¼ teaspoon alcohol-free vanilla extract
½ cup Brown Sugar Peach Topping
   (page 144), cooled

1. In a small bowl, whisk the yogurt, honey, and vanilla together.

2. In two parfait dishes, layer the yogurt with alternating layers of peach topping. Serve immediately.

tip Chop 2 tablespoons pecans and sprinkle them over the top of the parfaits for texture and added flavor.

PER SERVING (1 parfait) Calories: 321; Total Fat: 14g; Saturated Fat: 8g; Cholesterol: 14mg; Carbohydrates: 37g; Fiber: 0g; Protein: 11; Sodium: 163mg

Fruit Skewers *with* Honey Yogurt Dip

ALKALINE **GLUTEN-FREE** VEGETARIAN

Makes 6 skewers
Prep: 15 minutes

Fruit skewers make a simple and tasty snack that are great for picnics, potlucks, or just as a yummy snack on the go—and kids love them, too! This recipe doesn't involve any cooking, so it comes together in a snap.

2 cups cantaloupe balls
2 cups honeydew melon balls
2 cups watermelon balls
1½ cups nonfat plain Greek-style yogurt
3 tablespoons honey
1 teaspoon ground cinnamon

1. Using 6 skewers, thread each with the cantaloupe, honeydew, and watermelon.

2. In a small bowl, whisk the yogurt, honey, and cinnamon together.

3. Serve the skewers with the yogurt dip.

tip This works best with soft fruits like melons, but you can also use apples or pears for a little crunch.

PER SERVING (2 skewers with ¼ cup dip)
Calories: 120; Total Fat: <1g; Saturated Fat: 0g; Cholesterol: 1mg; Carbohydrates: 27g; Fiber: 1g; Protein: 5g; Sodium: 67mg

Easy Pepitas

ALKALINE GLUTEN-FREE LOW-CARB PALEO VEGAN

Serves 6
Prep: 5 minutes
Cook: 13 minutes

Pepitas, or hulled pumpkin seeds, make a healthy and tasty snack. They are loaded with healthy omega-3 fatty acids. While they are a little higher in fat, if you maintain portion control, they won't trigger your acid reflux.

6 ounces raw pepitas
2 tablespoons extra-virgin olive oil
¼ teaspoon sea salt

1. Preheat the oven to 325°F.

2. Line a baking sheet with parchment paper.

3. In a small bowl, toss the pepitas with the oil and salt. Spread into a single layer on the prepared sheet.

4. Bake for about 13 minutes until fragrant and starting to brown. Serve warm or cooled.

tip Sweeten your pepitas by replacing the salt with 2 tablespoons sugar and ¼ teaspoon ground cinnamon.

PER SERVING (1 ounce) Calories: 193; Total Fat: 17g; Saturated Fat: 3g; Cholesterol: 0mg; Carbohydrates: 6g; Fiber: 1g; Protein: 7g; Sodium: 83mg

Easy Vanilla Pudding

GLUTEN-FREE VEGAN

Serves 6
Prep: 5 minutes
Cook: 5 minutes
Chill: 20 minutes to 1 hour

Many people don't realize how easy it is to make homemade pudding. It takes about 10 minutes from start to finish, and the result tastes so much better than the stuff that comes in a box. You'll need to refrigerate the pudding for about an hour before serving, unless you like your pudding warm. You can do this more quickly in the freezer if you can't wait.

3 cups plain nondairy milk, divided
½ cup sugar
3 tablespoons cornstarch
1 teaspoon alcohol-free vanilla extract
¼ teaspoon sea salt

1. In a medium saucepan over medium heat, combine 2½ cups of milk and the sugar. Cook for about 3 minutes, stirring constantly until the mixture boils.

2. In a small bowl, whisk the cornstarch and remaining ½ cup of milk together. Stir this into the boiling pudding. Return to a boil and cook for 1 minute more, stirring constantly.

3. Stir in the vanilla and salt.

4. Refrigerate for about an hour before serving, or spoon the pudding into six (4-ounce) ramekins and freeze for 20 minutes.

tip To make this paleo, replace the milk with almond milk, the sugar with an equal amount of honey, and the cornstarch with 3 tablespoons arrowroot powder.

PER SERVING (½ cup) Calories: 125; Total Fat: 0g; Saturated Fat: 0g; Cholesterol: 0mg; Carbohydrates: 26g; Fiber: 0g; Protein: 4g; Sodium: 143mg

Butterscotch Pudding

VEGETARIAN

Serves 4
Prep: 10 minutes
Cook: 10 minutes
Chill: 20 minutes to 1 hour

Butterscotch pudding is one of those desserts that just feels like getting a big hug from Grandma. It's great warm or chilled, but truth be told, when my boys were small they would fight to lick the pan, and the pudding never made it until it was cooled.

2 tablespoons unsalted butter
½ cup packed dark brown sugar
2 cups skim milk
3 tablespoons cornstarch
1 teaspoon alcohol-free vanilla extract
¼ teaspoon sea salt

1. In a medium saucepan over medium-high heat, melt the butter and brown sugar until they simmer.

2. In a small bowl, whisk the milk and cornstarch together until smooth. Pour this slowly into the brown sugar mixture, whisking constantly, and bring to a simmer. Reduce the heat to medium-low. Simmer for about 2 minutes, whisking constantly until the pudding thickens.

3. Whisk in the vanilla and salt.

4. Spoon evenly into four (6-ounce) ramekins and chill until ready to serve.

tip To make this lactose-free or vegan, replace the milk with an equal amount of plain almond milk or rice milk.

PER SERVING (½ cup) Calories: 191; Total Fat: 6g; Saturated fat: 4g; Sodium: 229mg; Carbohydrates: 29g; Fiber: 0g; Protein: 4g; Sodium: 143mg

Chia Pudding

ALKALINE **PALEO** VEGAN

Serves 4
Prep: 15 minutes
Chill: 4 hours

Chia is a great source of omega-3 fatty acids. When it is soaked in liquid, it turns into gel-like globes similar to the texture of tapioca, perfect for a healthy, quick, no-cook pudding. It is so tasty and easy to make, I'll bet it will become a regular part of your rotation.

2 cups unsweetened almond milk
½ cup chia seeds
¼ cup pure maple syrup
1 teaspoon alcohol-free vanilla extract
½ teaspoon ground cinnamon
Pinch sea salt
1 banana, sliced (optional)

1. In a small bowl, whisk together the almond milk, chia seeds, maple syrup, vanilla, cinnamon, and salt.

2. Refrigerate for at least 4 hours.

3. Spoon into bowls and top with banana slices (if using).

tip You can also make a less lumpy version of this by puréeing all the ingredients in a blender before refrigerating.

PER SERVING (½ cup) Calories: 215; Total Fat: 6g; Saturated Fat: <1g; Cholesterol: 0mg; Carbohydrates: 37g; Fiber: 5g; Protein: 3g; Sodium: 83mg

Bananas Foster

Serves 4
Prep: 5 minutes
Cook: 11 minutes

Hands down, Bananas Foster is my favorite dessert ever. I'd rather have it than anything chocolate. I just love the warm caramel flavor of the sauce with the slight hint of cinnamon and creamy bananas. Delicious! This version eliminates the rum, but still has the same basic flavor profile.

3 tablespoons unsalted butter
2 bananas, sliced
¼ cup packed brown sugar
1 teaspoon ground cinnamon
Pinch sea salt
¼ cup apple juice
2 cups fat-free frozen vanilla yogurt

1. In a large sauté pan or skillet over medium-high heat, melt the butter until it bubbles.

2. Add the bananas, brown sugar, cinnamon, and salt. Cook for about 10 minutes, stirring constantly until the bananas caramelize.

3. Stir in the apple juice.

4. Serve warm over the frozen yogurt.

tip If you like the rummy flavor of the original Bananas Foster, add ½ teaspoon alcohol-free rum extract to the apple juice.

PER SERVING (½ cup frozen yogurt plus ¼ cup sauce) Calories: 262; Total Fat: 11g; Saturated Fat: 7g; Cholesterol: 28mg; Carbohydrates: 45g; Fiber: 5g; Protein: 4g; Sodium: 130mg

Butterscotch Sundaes

GLUTEN-FREE VEGETARIAN

Serves 4
Prep: 5 minutes
Cook: 10 minutes

Butterscotch is easy to make—it's just a combination of butter and dark brown sugar with a touch of dairy. Keep the fat low by consuming small portions, and eat it slowly to truly savor the sweet, salty taste of delicious butterscotch on creamy vanilla ice cream.

3 tablespoons unsalted butter
½ cup packed dark brown sugar
2 tablespoons pure maple syrup
¼ cup skim milk
2 tablespoons heavy (whipping) cream
Pinch sea salt
2 cups low-fat vanilla ice cream

1. In a medium saucepan over medium-high heat, melt the butter until it bubbles.

2. Add the brown sugar and maple syrup and cook for about 6 minutes, stirring constantly until the sugar has dissolved and the mixture boils.

3. Stir in the milk, heavy cream, and salt. Cook for 2 minutes more, stirring constantly.

4. Serve spooned over the ice cream.

tip Sprinkle each sundae with 1 tablespoon chopped peanuts for added texture.

PER SERVING (½ cup ice cream plus 2 tablespoons sauce) Calories: 271; Total Fat: 15g; Saturated Fat: 9g; Cholesterol: 48mg; Carbohydrates: 34g; Fiber: 0g; Protein: 2g; Sodium: 144mg

Banana Ice Cream

GLUTEN-FREE LOW-FODMAP PALEO VEGAN

Serves 6
Prep: 5 minutes

This recipe is so simple it's almost criminal. The result is a creamy frozen treat so full of flavor you'll be shocked it only took you five minutes to make in your blender. Eat it plain, topped with Brown Sugar Peach Topping (page 144) or Butterscotch (see page 160). You can't go wrong with this easy recipe.

3 bananas, peeled, sliced, and frozen
Pinch ground nutmeg

1. Place the frozen bananas in a blender or food processor. Add the nutmeg.

2. Blend until smooth, about 5 minutes.

tip For a creamier ice cream, add 2 tablespoons heavy (whipping) cream to the blender with the bananas.

PER SERVING (¼ cup) Calories: 53; Total Fat: 0g; Saturated Fat: 0g; Cholesterol: 0mg; Carbohydrates: 14g; Fiber: 2g; Protein: <1g; Sodium: 1mg

Caramel Apple Sundaes

GLUTEN-FREE VEGETARIAN

Serves 4
Prep: 10 minutes
Cook: 11 minutes

I love the flavor of cooked apples, especially when they are cooked with warming sweet spices like cinnamon and nutmeg. If you love caramel apples but hate how difficult they are to bite, you'll enjoy this version because it's easy on the teeth—and the stomach.

2 tablespoons unsalted butter
2 red apples, peeled, cored, and cut into ¼-inch dice
¼ cup pure maple syrup
½ cup packed dark brown sugar
1 teaspoon ground cinnamon
¼ teaspoon ground nutmeg
¼ teaspoon ground ginger
¼ teaspoon sea salt
2 tablespoons heavy (whipping) cream
2 cups low-fat vanilla ice cream

1. In a large sauté pan or skillet over medium-high heat, melt the butter until it bubbles.

2. Add the apples. Cook for about 5 minutes, stirring occasionally until they start to soften.

3. Add the maple syrup, brown sugar, cinnamon, nutmeg, ginger, and salt. Cook for 5 minutes more, stirring occasionally.

4. Stir in the heavy cream. Serve the sauce spooned over the ice cream.

tip Top each sundae with 2 tablespoons Cinnamon Granola (page 37) for some crunch.

PER SERVING (½ cup ice cream with ¼ cup topping) Calories: 326; Total Fat: 12g; Saturated Fat: 8g; Cholesterol: 40mg; Carbohydrates: 55g; Fiber: 3g; Protein: 2g; Sodium: 195mg

Pumpkin Mousse

ALKALINE   VEGETARIAN

Serves 8
Prep: 10 minutes

This creamy pumpkin mousse is a delicious, light dessert. It makes use of the Easy Vanilla Pudding on page 156 and includes a little bit of whipped cream, so keep your portions small so you don't aggravate your acid reflux with too much fat.

3 cups (1 recipe) Easy Vanilla Pudding (page 156)

1 (15-ounce) can pumpkin purée

2 tablespoons pure maple syrup

1 teaspoon pumpkin pie spice

1 cup whipped cream

1. In a large bowl, stir together the pudding, pumpkin purée, maple syrup, and pumpkin pie spice until well mixed.

2. Fold in the whipped cream.

tip For a richer mousse, you can also use Butterscotch Pudding (page 157) in place of the vanilla pudding.

PER SERVING (½ cup) Calories: 169;
Total Fat: 5g; Saturated Fat: 3g; Cholesterol: 18mg;
Carbohydrates: 28g; Fiber: 2g; Protein: 4g;
Sodium: 161mg

Crispy Rice Treats
with White Chocolate Chips

ALKALINE

Serves 8
Prep: 10 minutes
Cook: 5 minutes

Remember Rice Krispies treats? These are still as delicious, although they get a bit of a grown-up makeover with the addition of white chocolate chips. The gooey marshmallows and crispy rice will take you right back to the flavors of childhood.

Nonstick cooking spray
2 tablespoons unsalted butter
1 cup mini marshmallows
6 cups crisped rice cereal
1 cup white chocolate chips

1. Spray a 9-inch-square baking pan with nonstick cooking spray.

2. In a large pot over medium heat, melt the butter and marshmallows, stirring constantly until melted, about 5 minutes.

3. Stir in the cereal and white chocolate chips.

4. Spread in the prepared pan and let cool.

tip Looking for a fun flavor? Add 1 cup crushed banana chips (dried bananas) in place of the white chocolate chips. To make it vegetarian, use vegetarian marshmallows instead.

PER SERVING (1 treat) Calories: 174; Total Fat: 10g; Saturated Fat: 6g; Cholesterol: 12mg; Carbohydrates: 21g; Fiber: 0g; Protein: 1g; Sodium: 45mg

Banana Pudding Parfaits

ALKALINE   VEGETARIAN

Serves 6
Prep: 10 minutes

This is another dessert you can make using Easy Vanilla Pudding (page 156). With creamy pudding, flavorful bananas, and the nice crunch of low-fat vanilla wafers, this is a lovely and easy-to-make dessert.

2 bananas, peeled and sliced
3 cups (1 recipe) Easy Vanilla Pudding (page 156)
12 vanilla wafers, crushed into crumbs
6 tablespoons whipped cream

1. In each of 6 parfait dishes, place a layer of bananas followed by a layer of pudding followed by a layer of wafer crumbs. Repeat.

2. Top each with 1 tablespoon of whipped cream.

tip To crush the cookies, place them in a zip-top bag, seal, and hit the bag with a rolling pin or can.

PER SERVING (1 parfait) Calories: 239;
Total Fat: 6g; Saturated Fat: 3g; Cholesterol: 23mg;
Carbohydrates: 41g; Fiber: 1g; Protein: 5g;
Sodium: 173mg

White Chocolate Truffles

ALKALINE   VEGETARIAN

Makes 8
Prep: 5 minutes
Cook: 10 minutes
Chill: 20 minutes

What could be a more perfect bite to finish off a meal than a decadent white chocolate truffle? The key here is portion control. Limit yourself to one truffle to keep your fat low. These truffles are so satisfying, one is all you'll need.

4 ounces white chocolate chips
½ cup nonfat plain Greek-style yogurt
¼ cup powdered sugar

1. In a double boiler, melt the white chocolate chips, stirring constantly.

2. Remove from the heat and stir in the yogurt.

3. Freeze the mixture for about 20 minutes or until firm.

4. Pour the powdered sugar onto a plate.

5. Divide the truffle mixture into 8 pieces and roll each into a ball. Roll in the powdered sugar to coat.

tip If you don't have a double boiler, don't sweat it. You can either place a glass bowl in a pan of water with the bottom just above the water, or heat the white chocolate in the microwave in 30-second increments, stirring every 30 seconds until melted.

PER SERVING (1 truffle) Calories: 100; Total Fat: 5g; Saturated Fat: 3g; Cholesterol: 3mg; Carbohydrates: 13g; Fiber: 0g; Protein: 2g; Sodium: 25mg

White Chocolate–Dipped Strawberries

GLUTEN-FREE VEGETARIAN

Serves 4
Prep: 10 minutes
Chill: 10 minutes

If you're looking for an easy and elegant sweet treat, dipping strawberries in white chocolate is a great way to go. The milky sweetness of the white chocolate complements the sweet, juicy strawberry flavor, and making this dessert is ridiculously easy. You can make the dessert more festive by dipping the coated strawberries in candy sprinkles, if you wish.

3 ounces white chocolate, chopped
12 large strawberries

1. Line a baking sheet with parchment paper.

2. In a small bowl set over a saucepan of barely simmering water, melt the white chocolate, stirring constantly until the chocolate has melted and is smooth. Remove the bowl from the heat.

3. Holding one strawberry by the stem, dip two-thirds of the strawberry into the melted white chocolate. Shake the strawberry gently to allow excess chocolate to drip off. Place the coated strawberry on the parchment-lined sheet to set. Repeat with the remaining strawberries.

4. Freeze the strawberries for 5 to 10 minutes to allow the chocolate to set before serving.

PER SERVING (4 dipped strawberries) Calories: 126; Total fat: 7g; Saturated fat: 4g; Cholesterol: 4mg; Carbohydrates: 15g; Fiber: <1g; Protein: 2g; Sodium: 19mg

tip You can also use a microwave to melt white chocolate. Place the white chocolate in a microwave-safe glass bowl and heat it at medium power (50 percent power) for 30 seconds. Stir the chocolate and heat again at medium power for 30 more seconds. Repeat this process until the chocolate is melted.

The FDA's pH Food List

The chart at the end of this appendix offers information from the Food and Drug Administration of the pH of various foods. You can use this list as a handy reference when planning your own acid reflux–friendly meals, so you're not just limited to the recipes available in this cookbook.

A LITTLE ABOUT PH

So what is pH? It's a measure of the acidity of a substance. Recalling from basic high school chemistry, substances fall on a scale of acidity and alkalinity, known as the pH scale. A pH of 7 indicates a substance is neutral—that is, it has no acidity or alkalinity. For example, water tends to hover around a pH of 7, although it is possible to find both acid and alkaline waters, so the range is more like 6.5 to 8.5.

Substances with a pH *below* 7 are acidic. The lower the number, the more acidic the substance is. For each whole number you drop, acidity increases by 10 times. So something with a pH of 6 is 10 times more acidic than something with a pH of 7; something with a pH of 5 is 100 times more acidic, and so on.

Substances with a pH *above* 7 are alkaline, and alkalinity increases 10 times per each whole number it goes up. Baking soda has an alkalinity of around 8, which means it is 10 times more alkaline than water. The most alkaline substances, like lye, have an alkalinity of 14, making them highly caustic.

PH AND YOUR BODY

Your body has a pH range from 7.3 to 7.5, so it is slightly alkaline, although pH levels vary throughout your different body parts. Your stomach is, by nature, a highly acidic environment with a pH level of about 2.0. It needs to be, because hydrochloric acid (HCL) is essential for breaking down foods for the process of digestion. This pH level is 100,000 times more acidic than water. That's why stomach acid burns when it splashes into your throat, and why it can damage the delicate tissue in your esophagus.

PH AND FOOD

Foods tend to have a pH range from about 2 (for vinegar, or 2.2 for lemon juice) up to about 8.5 (found in some processed and baked goods), although most vegetables and legumes fall in a range of about 6.5 to about 7.5.

According to Dr. Jamie Kaufman, when dealing with acid reflux, you should select foods with a lower degree of acidity. It's important to minimize acidity in your stomach so it does less damage if it splashes into the esophagus. And eating foods with a higher pH can help reduce the acid in the stomach and thus minimize damage.

When selecting foods from these charts, keep the following in mind:

- If you have severe acid reflux or are just starting to heal, select foods with a pH of 5 or higher.

- If your acid reflux isn't as severely reactive, or if you've spent three months or more healing, you can probably select foods with a pH of 4 or higher.

- Adjust based on your own sensitivity. Test foods in different pH levels to determine what your threshold is for acidity in foods.

THE FDA'S PH FOOD LIST

VEGETABLES	PH
Artichokes, canned	5.7 to 6.0
Artichokes, fresh	5.6
Asparagus, canned	5.2 to 5.3
Asparagus, fresh	6.1 to 6.7
Beans, green	4.6
Beans, lima	6.5
Beets, canned	4.9
Beets, fresh	4.9 to 5.6
Brussels sprouts	6.0 to 6.3
Cabbage, green	5.4 to 6.9
Cabbage, red	5.4 to 6.0
Cabbage, savoy	6.3
Cabbage, white	6.2
Carrots, canned	5.2
Carrots, fresh	4.9 to 5.2
Cauliflower	5.6
Celery	5.7 to 6.0
Corn, canned	6.0
Corn, fresh	6.0 to 7.5
Cucumbers	5.1 to 5.7
Cucumbers, pickled	3.2 to 3.5

Eggplant	4.5 to 5.3
Hominy	6.0
Kale	6.4 to 6.8
Kohlrabi	5.7 to 5.8
Leeks	5.5 to 6.0
Lettuce	5.8 to 6.0
Mushrooms	6.2
Okra	5.5 to 6.4
Olives, black	6.0 to 6.5
Olives, green	3.6 to 3.8
Onions, red	5.3 to 5.8
Onions, white	5.4 to 5.8
Onions, yellow	5.4 to 5.6
Parsnips	5.3
Peas, canned	5.7 to 6.0
Peas, fresh	5.8 to 7.0
Peas, frozen	6.4 to 6.7
Peppers, bell	5.2
Potatoes, russet	6.1
Potatoes, sweet	5.3 to 5.6
Pumpkin	4.8 to 5.2
Radishes, red	5.8 to 6.5
Radishes, white	5.5 to 5.7

Rhubarb	3.1 to 3.4
Sauerkraut	3.5 to 3.6
Spinach, fresh	5.5 to 6.8
Spinach, frozen	6.3 to 6.5
Squash	5.5 to 6.0
Tomatoes, canned	3.5 to 4.7
Tomatoes, fresh	4.2 to 4.9
Tomato juice	4.1 to 4.2
Tomato paste	3.5 to 4.7
Turnips	5.2 to 5.5
Zucchini	5.8 to 6.1

GRAINS & LEGUMES	PH
Beans, kidney	5.4 to 6.0
Bread	5.3 to 5.8
Cake	5.2 to 8.0
Crackers	7.0 to 8.5
Flour	6.0 to 6.3
Lentils	6.3 to 6.8
Rice, brown	6.2 to 6.7
Rice, white	6.0 to 6.7
Rice, wild	6.0 to 6.4

HERBS	PH
Chives	5.2 to 6.1
Horseradish	5.35
Parsley	5.7 to 6.0
Sorrel	3.7

DAIRY	PH
Butter	6.1 to 6.4
Buttermilk	4.5
Milk	6.3 to 8.5
Cream	6.5
Cheese, Camembert	7.4
Cheese, Cheddar	5.9
Cheese, cottage	5.0
Cheese, cream	4.9
Cheese, Edam	5.4
Cheese, Roquefort	5.5 to 5.9
Cheese, Swiss	5.1 to 6.6
Eggs, whites	7.0 to 9.0
Eggs, whole	7.1 to 7.9
Eggs, yolks	6.4

FRUITS	PH			
Apples	3.3 to 3.9		Nectarines	3.9
Apple juice	3.4 to 4.0		Oranges	3.1 to 4.1
Applesauce	3.3 to 3.6		Orange juice	3.6 to 4.3
Apricots, canned	3.7		Papaya	5.2 to 5.7
Apricots, dried	3.6 to 4.0		Peaches, canned	4.9
Apricots, fresh	3.3 to 4.0		Peaches, fresh	3.4 to 3.6
Bananas	4.5 to 5.2		Peaches, jarred	4.2
Blackberries	3.2 to 4.5		Persimmons	5.4 to 5.8
Blueberries, fresh	3.7		Pineapple, canned	3.5
Blueberries, frozen	3.1 to 3.4		Pineapple, fresh	3.3 to 5.2
Cantaloupe	6.2 to 7.1		Plums	2.8 to 4.6
Cherries	3.2 to 4.1		Pomegranates	3.0
Cranberry juice	2.3 to 2.5		Prunes	3.1 to 5.4
Cranberry sauce	2.4		Prune juice	3.7
Dates	6.3 to 6.6		Raspberries	3.2 to 3.7
Figs	4.6		Strawberries, fresh	3.0 to 3.5
Grapefruit	3.0 to 3.3		Strawberries, frozen	2.3 to 3.0
Grapes	3.4 to 4.5		Tangerines	4.0
Lemons	2.2 to 2.4		Watermelon	5.2 to 5.8
Limes	1.8 to 2.0			
Mango	3.9 to 4.6			
Melons, honeydew	6.3 to 6.7			

MEAT, POULTRY, FISH	PH
Beef, ground	5.1 to 6.2
Beef, steak	5.8 to 7.0
Chicken	6.5 to 6.7
Clams	6.5
Crab	7.0
Fish	6.6 to 7.3
Ham	5.9 to 6.1
Lamb	5.4 to 6.7
Oysters	4.8 to 6.3
Pork	5.3 to 6.9
Salmon	6.1 to 6.3
Shrimp	6.8 to 7.0
Tuna	5.2 to 6.1
Turkey	5.7 to 6.8
Veal	6.0
Whitefish	5.5

OTHER	PH
Cider	2.9 to 3.3
Cocoa	6.3
Corn syrup	5.0
Cornstarch	4.0 to 7.0
Ginger ale	2.0 to 4.0
Honey	3.9
Jam	3.1 to 3.5
Mayonnaise	4.2 to 4.5
Molasses	5.0 to 5.5
Raisins	3.8 to 4.0
Sugar	5.0 to 6.0
Vinegar	2.0 to 3.5
Yeast	3.0 to 3.5

Measurement Conversions

VOLUME EQUIVALENTS (LIQUID)

US STANDARD	US STANDARD (OUNCES)	METRIC (APPROXIMATE)
2 tablespoons	1 fl. oz.	30 mL
¼ cup	2 fl. oz.	60 mL
½ cup	4 fl. oz.	120 mL
1 cup	8 fl. oz.	240 mL
1½ cups	12 fl. oz.	355 mL
2 cups or 1 pint	16 fl. oz.	475 mL
4 cups or 1 quart	32 fl. oz.	1 L
1 gallon	128 fl. oz.	4 L

OVEN TEMPERATURES

FAHRENHEIT	CELSIUS (APPROXIMATE)
250°F	120°C
300°F	150°C
325°F	165°C
350°F	180°C
375°F	190°C
400°F	200°C
425°F	220°C
450°F	230°C

VOLUME EQUIVALENTS (DRY)

US STANDARD	METRIC (APPROXIMATE)
⅛ teaspoon	0.5 mL
¼ teaspoon	1 mL
½ teaspoon	2 mL
¾ teaspoon	4 mL
1 teaspoon	5 mL
1 tablespoon	15 mL
¼ cup	59 mL
⅓ cup	79 mL
½ cup	118 mL
⅔ cup	156 mL
¾ cup	177 mL
1 cup	235 mL
2 cups or 1 pint	475 mL
3 cups	700 mL
4 cups or 1 quart	1 L

WEIGHT EQUIVALENTS

US STANDARD	METRIC (APPROXIMATE)
½ ounce	15 g
1 ounce	30 g
2 ounces	60 g
4 ounces	115 g
8 ounces	225 g
12 ounces	340 g
16 ounces or 1 pound	455 g

The Dirty Dozen & The Clean Fifteen

A nonprofit environmental watchdog organization called Environmental Working Group (EWG) looks at data supplied by the US Department of Agriculture (USDA) and the Food and Drug Administration (FDA) about pesticide residues. Each year it compiles a list of the best and worst pesticide loads found in commercial crops. You can use these lists to decide which fruits and vegetables to buy organic to minimize your exposure to pesticides and which produce is considered safe enough to buy conventionally. This does not mean they are pesticide-free, though, so wash these fruits and vegetables thoroughly.

These lists change every year, so make sure you look up the most recent one before you fill your shopping cart. You'll find the most recent lists, as well as a guide to pesticides in produce, at EWG.org/FoodNews.

Dirty Dozen

Apples	Nectarines	*In addition to the Dirty Dozen, the EWG added two types of produce contaminated with highly toxic organophosphate insecticides:*
Celery	Peaches	
Cherries	Spinach	
Cherry tomatoes	Strawberries	
Cucumbers	Sweet bell peppers	Kale/Collard greens
Grapes	Tomatoes	Hot peppers

Clean Fifteen

Asparagus	Eggplant	Onions
Avocados	Grapefruit	Papayas
Cabbage	Honeydew Melon	Pineapples
Cantaloupe	Kiwis	Sweet corn
Cauliflower	Mangos	Sweet peas (frozen)

References

Amos, Julie-Ann. "Acid Reflux (GERD) Statistics and Facts." Healthline. June 30, 2012. Accessed November 13, 2016. www.healthline.com/health/gerd/statistics#2.

Bardot, Jean. "Ten Tips to Cure Acid Reflux Naturally." NaturalNews. Accessed November 13, 2016. www.naturalnews.com/034461_holidays_meals_acid_reflux.html.

Beyond Celiac. "Celiac Disease: Fast Facts." Accessed November 13, 2016. www.beyondceliac.org/celiac-disease/facts-and-figures.

Beyond Celiac. "Non-Celiac Gluten Sensitivity." Accessed November 13, 2016. www.beyondceliac.org/celiac-disease/non-celiac-gluten-sensitivity.

Cleveland Clinic. "Hiatal Hernia." Accessed November 13, 2016. http://my.clevelandclinic.org/health/diseases_conditions/hic-hernia/hic-hiatal-hernia.

Connealey, Leigh Erin. "How pH Levels and Acidity Relate to Heartburn." NaturalNews. June 27, 2008. Accessed November 13, 2016. www.naturalnews.com/023526_esophagus_heartburn_pH_levels.html.

Dent, J., H. B. El-Serag, M. A. Wallander, and S. Johansson. "Epidemiology of Gastro-Oesophageal Reflux Disease: A Systematic Review." *Gut* 54, no. 5 (May 2005): 710–717. doi:10.1136/gut.2004.051821.

Elmhurst University. "pH Scale." Virtual Chembook. Accessed November 13, 2016. http://chemistry.elmhurst.edu/vchembook/184ph.html.

Gardner, Amanda. "9 Medications That Can Cause Heartburn." Health.com. Accessed November 13, 2016. www.health.com/health/gallery/0,,20400680,00.html.

IFFGD. "Antacids." Last modified September 4, 2015. Accessed November 13, 2016. www.iffgd.org/diet-treatments/antacids.html.

Koufman, Jamie, Sonia Huang, and Philip Gelb. *Dr. Koufman's Acid Reflux Diet: 111 All New Reflux-Friendly Recipes, Including Vegan & Gluten-Free*. New York: Katalitix Media, 2015.

Kresser, Chris. "More Evidence to Support the Theory That GERD Is Caused by Bacterial Overgrowth." Chris Kresser. July 16, 2014. Accessed November 13, 2016. https://chriskresser.com/more-evidence-to-support-the-theory-that-gerd-is-caused-by-bacterial-overgrowth.

Kresser, Chris. "The Hidden Causes of Heartburn and GERD." Chris Kresser. Accessed November 13, 2016. https://chriskresser.com/the-hidden-causes-of-heartburn-and-gerd.

Levine, Arie, Svetlana Domanov, Igor Sukhotnik, Tsili Zangen, and Ron Shaoul. "Celiac-Associated Peptic Disease at Upper Endoscopy: How Common Is It?" *Scandinavian Journal of Gastroenterology* 44, no. 12 (November 2009): 1424–28. doi: 10.3109/00365520903307987.

Marcin, Ashley. "Can You Eat Dairy If You Have Acid Reflux?" Healthline. Accessed November 13, 2016. www.healthline.com/health/gerd/dairy-and-acid-reflux#Overview1.

Mayo Clinic. "Eosinophilic Esophagitis." Accessed November 13, 2016. www.mayoclinic.org/diseases-conditions/eosinophilic-esophagitis/basics/definition/con-20035681.

Mayo Clinic. "GERD." Accessed November 13, 2016. www.mayoclinic.org/diseasesconditions/gerd/basics/causes/con-20025201.

Monash University. "Low FODMAP Diet for Irritable Bowel Syndrome." Accessed November 13, 2016. www.med.monash.edu/cecs/gastro/fodmap.

National Institute of Diabetes and Digestive and Kidney Diseases. "Definition and Facts for GER and GERD." Accessed November 13, 2016. www.niddk.nih.gov/health-information/health-topics/digestive-diseases/ger-and-gerd-in-adults/Pages/definition-facts.aspx.

Panahi, Yunes, Hossein Khedmat, Ghasem Valizadegan, Reza Mohtashami, and Amirhossein Sahebkar. "Efficacy and Safety of Aloe Vera Syrup for the Treatment of Gastroesophageal Reflux Disease: A Pilot Randomized Positive-Controlled Trial." *Journal of Traditional Chinese Medicine* 35, no. 6 (December 2015): 632–36.

Peek, Richard M. "Helicobacter Pylori and Gastroesophageal Reflux Disease." *Current Treatment Options in Gastroenterology* 7, no. 1 (February 2004): 59–70. doi:10.1007/s11938-004-0026-0.

Richter, Joel E. "Advances in GERD: Current Developments in the Management of Acid-Related GI Disorders." *Gastroenterology & Hepatology*. New York: Millennium Medical Publishing, Inc., September 2009.

Song, Eun Mi, Hye-Kyung Jung, and Ji Min Jung. "The Association Between Reflux Esophagitis and Psychosocial Stress." *Digestive Diseases and Sciences* 58, no. 2 (February 2013): 471–77. doi:10.1007/s10620-012-2377-z.

Sugerman, Harvey J. "Increased Intra-Abdominal Pressure and GERD/Barrett's Esophagus." *Gastroenterology* 133, no. 6 (December 2007): 2075. doi:http://dx.doi.org/10.1053/j.gastro.2007.10.017.

US FDA. "BBB—pH Values of Various Foods." *pH Values of Various Foods.* Accessed November 13, 2016. www.fda.gov/Food/FoodborneIllnessContaminants/CausesOfIllnessBadBugBook/ucm122561.htm.

US National Library of Medicine. "Aging Changes in the Bones, Muscles, Joints." Medline Plus. Accessed November 13, 2016. https://medlineplus.gov/ency/article/004015.htm.

Williams, David. "Natural Treatments and Remedies for Acid Reflux." Dr. David Williams. Accessed November 13, 2016. www.drdavidwilliams.com/acid-reflux-natural-treatments.

Resources

BOOKS

Frazier, Karen. *Acid Reflux Escape Plan: Two Weeks to Heartburn Relief*. Sonoma Press: August, 2015.

Koufman, Jamie. *Dr. Koufman's Acid Reflux Diet*. Katalitix: December, 2015.

Koufman, Jamie, Jordan Stern, and Marc Michael Bauer. *Dropping Acid: The Reflux Diet Cookbook & Cure*. Reflux Cookbooks: September, 2010.

WEBSITES

American College of Gastroenterology Acid Reflux: http://patients.gi.org/topics /acid-reflux/

Dr. Jamie Koufman's website: www.voiceinstituteofnewyork.com

FDA. pH values of various foods: www.fda.gov/Food/FoodborneIllness Contaminants/CausesOfIllnessBad BugBook/ucm122561.htm

Monash University Low-FODMAP website: www.med.monash.edu/cecs/gastro /fodmap/low-high.html

APPS

Acid Reflux Diet Food Checker by Joanne Gelato: https://itunes.apple.com/us/app /acid-reflux-diet/id686398462?mt=8

Fast Tract Diet App for Gut Health by the Digestive Health Institute: https://digestivehealthinstitute.org /2015/12/17/fast-tract-diet-app/

GERD, Heartburn, and Acid Reflux App: https://play.google.com/store/apps /details?id=com.GERDHeartburnand AcidRefluxSymptomsRemedies.app&hl=en

Monash University Low-FODMAP Diet App by Monash University: www.med.monash.edu.au/cecs/gastro /fodmap/iphone-app.html

Recipe Index

Index

Acknowledgments

Without my kitchen mentors—my mom, Brenda Riseland, and my other mom, Etta Kirk—I wouldn't have discovered my love for cooking, so for them I am very grateful. I'm also grateful for my food testers: my sons, Tanner Koenen and Kevin Frazier, my husband, Jim Frazier, and the many others I frequently push my food on. Thanks also to my editor, Clara Song Lee, who is a joy to work with.

CPSIA information can be obtained
at www.ICGtesting.com
Printed in the USA
LVHW022239081020
668299LV00004BA/7